21 DAYS

TO CHANGE YOUR LIFESTYLE HABITS

ISABELLE LIPARI

First Edition – 2014

Publications Mellifera

© All right reserved 2014

ISBN 978-2-9814451-2-4

Legal deposit – National Library and Archives of Quebec – 2014
Legal deposit – Library and Archives Canada – 2014

Scientific research: Science students Alexandre Fredette and Julia Lipari-Couture
Editing and proofreading: Julia Lipari-Couture and Maryse Lipari-Simms
Translation from French to English: Adam Lague
Graphic design: Nicole Reyes
Graphics for English version: Claude Dumont, Studio 42
Marketing and communications: Pierre G. Couture

For permission to use material from this text or product, contact us at:
514-426-6247 · info@aveolancis.com

This book was written to provide a simple and easy method to change lifestyle
habits. It does not replace, by any means whatsoever, a medical opinion or
treatment. It is up to the reader to judge his or her own medical condition and
to consult a health care professional if necessary.

"This book is dedicated to my mother, Francine Blain, who courageously battled cancer for more than six years. Her premature death has modeled the woman, wife, and mother that I have become."

Isabelle Lipari

TABLE OF CONTENTS

SECTION 1 NUTRITION

SECTION 2 PHYSICAL ACTIVITY

SECTION 3 STRESS MANAGEMENT AND WELLNESS

SECTION 4 SLEEP

APPENDICES

PREFACE

Our health is our most valuable asset. It's the condition that allows us to achieve our dreams, reach our goals, and maintain meaningful relationships with the people around us. It is our physical and psychological well-being that allows us to enjoy and benefit from every moment that life offers us.

But our health, which we so often take for granted, depends a large part on our lifestyle habits. It is often said: "It is easy to pick up bad habits, but difficult to live with their consequences, which often result in disease. On the other hand, it is often difficult to develop good habits, but easy to live with their consequences; namely, good health, energy, and well-being."

The author has done a remarkable job; and as a result the book you are holding offers quality information that is scientifically substantiated and presented in a way that is accessible and easy to understand. Although the method she is proposing will require some effort on your part, the path toward your final destination has been clearly articulated. Her method will allow you to gradually integrate healthier lifestyle habits into your life with ease. These habits will enable you to solidify your health and improve the quality of your life and the lives of your loved ones.

Mario Messier, M.D.
Medical Consultant in Workplace Health and Health Promotion
Scientific Director of The Healthy Enterprises Group
Medical Consultant in Workplace Health at Institut National de la santé publique du Québec

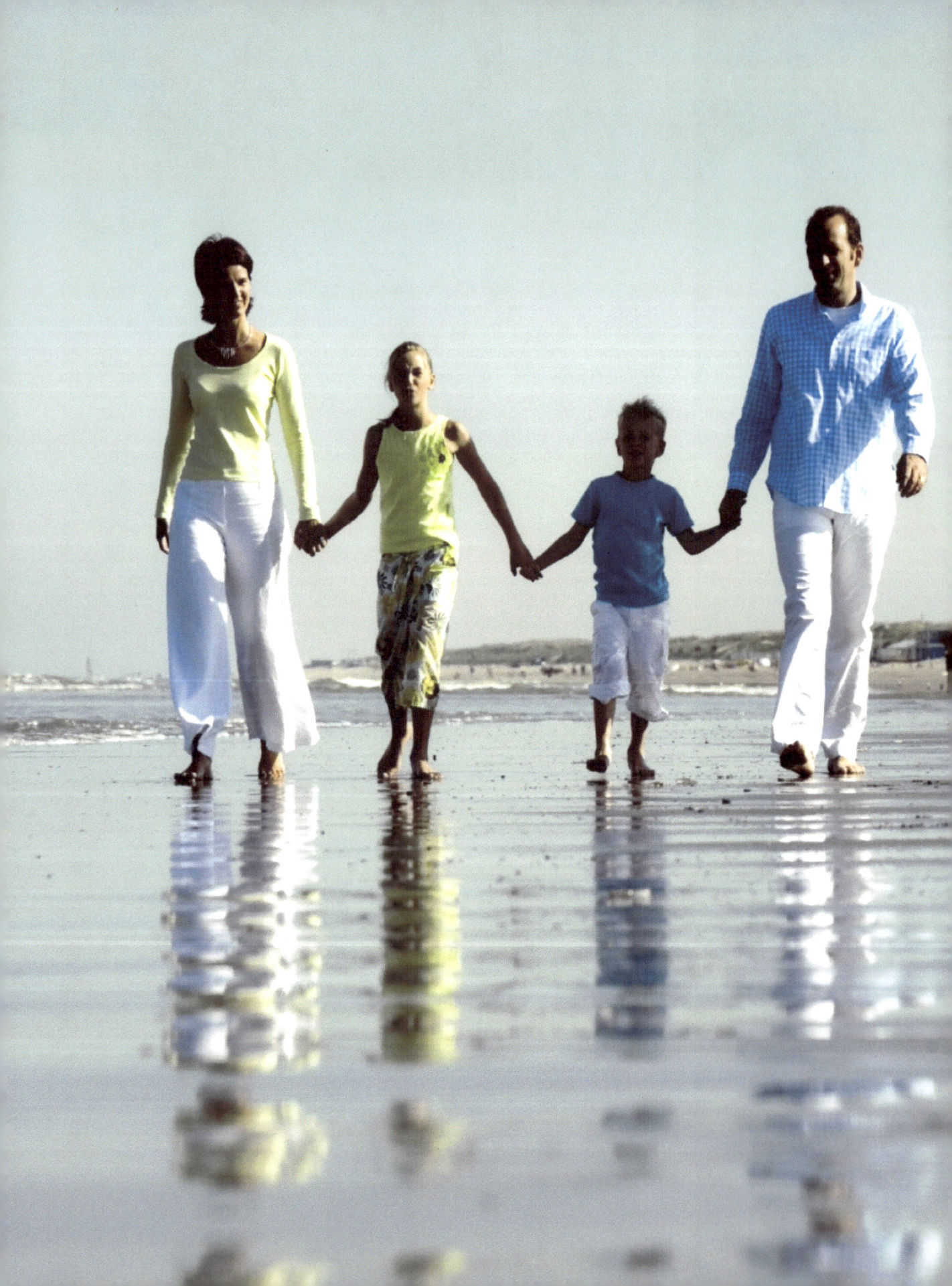

WHY 21 DAYS?

The idea that a habit can be changed in 21 days comes from the book Psycho-Cybernetics, written in 1960 by the cosmetic surgeon Dr. Maxwell Maltz. Dr. Maltz specialized in reconstruction and facial cosmetic surgery. He focused on the psychology of self-image and believed that improving self-image had to be triggered by an internal change.

After having done extensive research on patients that underwent facial reconstructions or amputations, Dr. Maltz found that it took at least 21 days for the patient to notice physical change. Patients with an amputated limb stopped undergoing the effects of phantom limb after a minimum of 21 days. He therefore concluded that to reprogram neurological pathways, it took a minimum of 21 days. He then applied this theory to habit changes to help his patients change their image, their thought process and daily habits.

More than 50 years after it was published, Psycho-Cybernetics is still considered one of the best self-improvement tools by Tom Butler-Bowdon in his 2008 work, 50 Self-Help Classics.

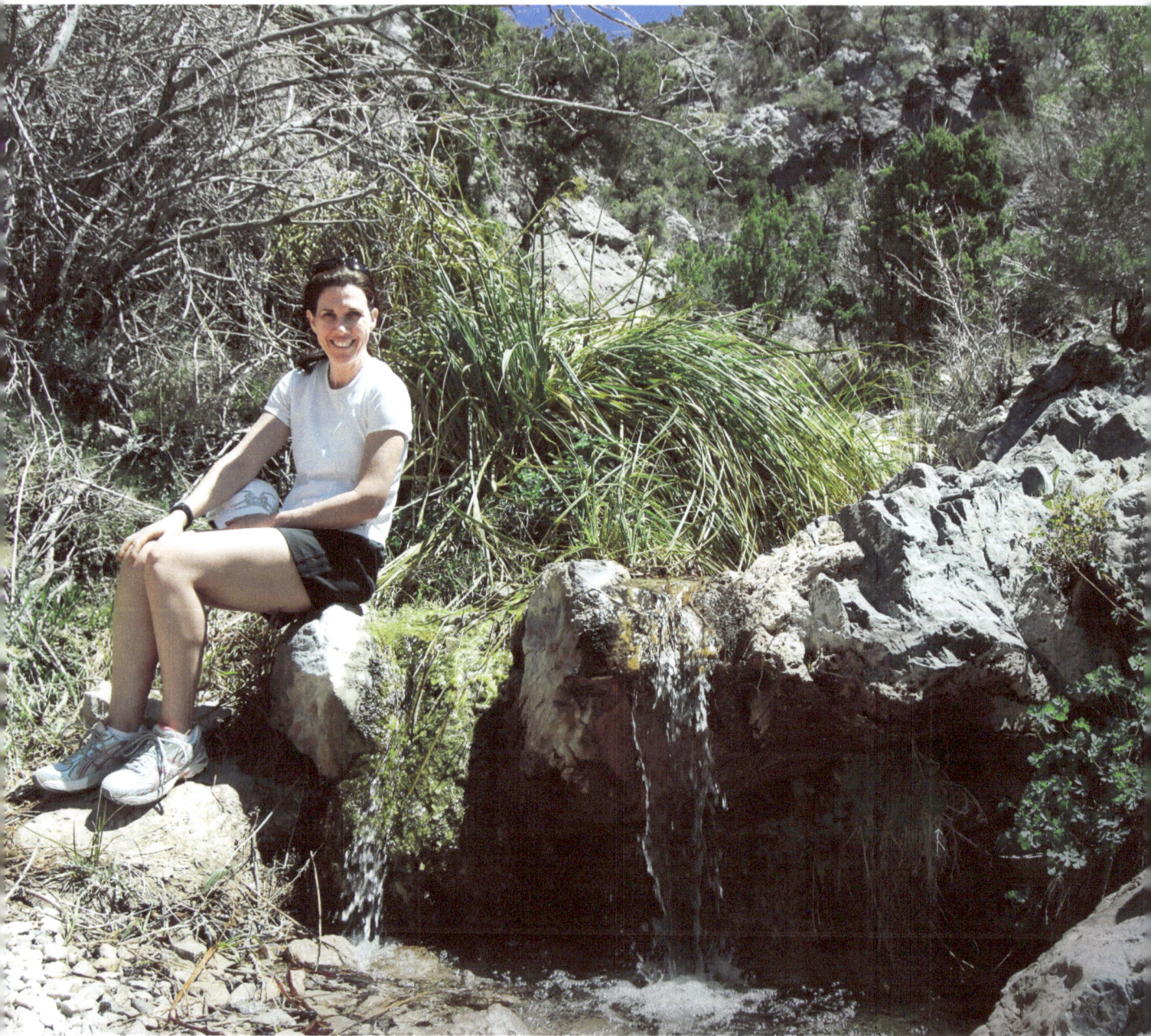

ABOUT THE AUTHOR

Isabelle Lipari has a degree in Business Administration, she is a certified personal trainer and a nutrition and wellness specialist. In 2007, she founded Aveolancis Corporate Health, whose mission is to promote health and wellness within companies.

Through the health programs she is implementing, she hopes to transmit her personal and professional experiences to people. Her own life journey has given her an appreciation for life, health, and happiness.

When Isabelle was only two years old, her mother was diagnosed with breast cancer. She underwent a mastectomy, hysterectomy, and several brain surgeries over the course of six years. At the young age of 39, she died of multiple brain metastases. Her family is a carrier of BRCA1 and BRCA2 genes. Four of her five sisters were diagnosed, as well as her mother and two aunts. All of them passed away except for two of her sisters who are still alive to this day.

On her father's side, Isabelle's godmother, uncle, and grandfather died of cardiovascular diseases. All of these deaths occurred before Isabelle was 15 years old. At such a young age, Isabelle was heavily affected by all these illnesses. She quickly became aware of the necessity of taking her health into her own hands, knowing her genetics were not favourable.

Despite this, at the age of 30, Isabelle was diagnosed with a malignant melanoma, the worst type of skin cancer. Fortunately it was detected in time. In 2007, her sister was diagnosed with breast cancer. She has passed the critical five-year period. In the fall of 2011, Isabelle's daughter was diagnosed with thyroid cancer. Several months later, she underwent a full thyroidectomy. She has recovered slowly, but her life has been changed forever...

In 50 years of life, Isabelle has seen several people close to her become ill or pass away. These hardships have defined her life.

Despite every sad event, she has succeeded in striking a balance, allowing herself to remain functional while happy. Married for more than 25 years, she and her husband have three wonderful children with whom they share life's best moments; those of happiness and joy.

These experiences are the reason Aveolancis − Corporate Health was created. Its objective is to promote health and healthy lifestyle habits to Quebecers. Isabelle is convinced that small changes made today, will lead to a better health and quality of life tomorrow.

Disease does not follow a criterion of age, sex, or race. It strikes unexpectedly, and it does not only affect the person it hits, but everyone around them as well.

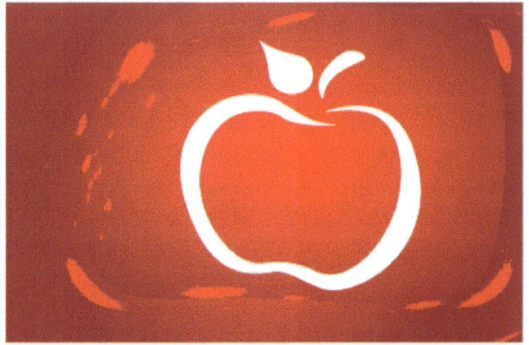

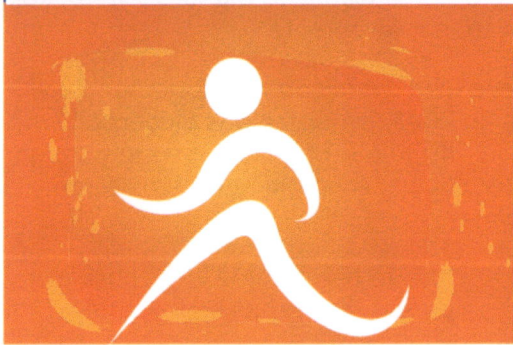

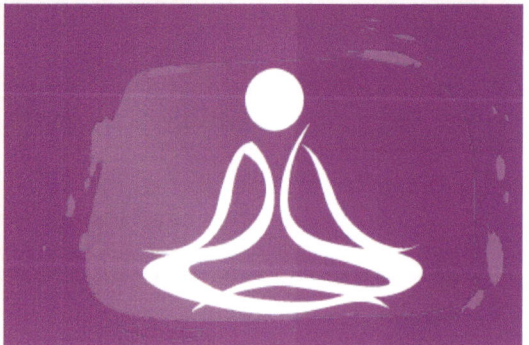

WHY WAS THIS GUIDE CREATED?

This guide was created to help people change their lifestyle habits, one at a time, by facilitating behaviour changes. It offers a simple and easy method to pick up healthy life habits that will impact the individual's health and quality of life.

The guide is not intended to be a diet or special weight loss program. Its content is based on basic medical and scientific data fundamental to maintaining a healthy body and mind. By adopting the 30 proposed habits set out in this guide, you reduce your risk of disease, increase your chances of living a longer life, and improve your quality of life.

Why improve these lifestyle habits? Because several studies have proved that poor lifestyle habits are responsible for 70% of cancers and 90% of heart diseases, the two most common causes of death in today's society.

While promoting healthy lifestyles in companies, the author found that people had a hard time changing habits that unfortunately had been rooted in their daily life for decades. Most of the advice offered in this guide has been inspired by the author's experience in consultation.

In general, people are resistant to change. They don't want to put in the effort necessary to make changes. Many need tremendous motivation or a notable experience to make a change in their life. There are countless stories of people that make drastic changes in their life only after having suffered a serious health problem. Why wait?

"Initiating a habit change is much easier when we are healthy, rather than in a state of sickness. Take charge of your health today," says the author.

This guide proposes an effective method, facilitating a lifestyle change with the help of precise steps and numerous tools available at the end of the book, or online in PDF format at aveolancis.com in the Publications section.

HOW TO USE THIS GUIDE

STEP 1

Browse the guide and identify habits you would like to change; those that apply to you. Choose the habit you would like to change in the next 21 days.

STEP 2

Choose a mentor or coach who can motivate you and will hold you accountable. He or she may support your commitment and help you stick to it. Together, you will decide the goal, some rewards, and penalties (see step 4).

STEP 3

The personal contract (appendix 1)

This document serves as a commitment to oneself. You will find it at the end of the book and online at aveolancis.com in the Publications section.

TIP

Start at an appropriate time, during your day off for example, when stress is at a minimum and you have time to fill out the documents, and undertake the required actions.

STEP 4

The 21-day logbook (Appendix 2 and 3)

This document serves as an action plan and contains all the necessary information in order to reach your goal.

1. Write down the habit you wish to change.
2. Turn your goal into a SMART* goal.
3. Identify the steps for success that will assure that you reach your goal.
4. Fill in the dates.
5. Sign the journal and identify one or more rewards.
6. Each day, use a checkmark to indicate success.

*See Appendix 4 for more information on how to create a SMART goal.

You can choose a reward every seven days or a bigger reward at the end of the 21 days. When choosing a reward, there are no limits. You can choose a treat, an outing, a purchase, or a trip. The goal is to choose something that makes you happy and motivates you.

After succeeding, you can move on to another habit, whenever the time is right.

OBJECTIF
SMART

S pecific

M easurable

A cceptable

R ealistic

T emporal

OPTIONAL STEP

Before starting, you may record your weight and waist size. You may also take a photo of yourself. Put the contract, your measurements, and the photo inside the page cover of this guide for your future reference.

Measurements: _____

Weight: _____

Waist size: _____

How to measure waist size: Take a measuring tape and place it just below your navel.

TIP

You will increase your chances of success if you keep a calendar within reach throughout the 21 days. If not, find a place for it where you can always see it, like on the fridge, on the bedside, or on the bulletin board. Remind yourself often of the actions you need to do to reach your goal.

STEP 5

Checkpoint no. 1 on day 7

It has already been a week since you have undertaken your transformation. It is time to take a break to confirm that you are on the right track. If you have ticked the box each of the seven days, you are on your way! And you can reward yourself.

If, on the other hand, you have had a hard time, begin the following steps:
1. Identify the context in which you haven't met your goals.
2. Write down the reasons you haven't made the changes.
3. Identify the reasons you've had difficulty.
4. Find possible solutions.
5. Determine the necessary actions to get back on track and readjust your plan of action.

Continue your efforts even if you haven't completely succeeded. It is possible that it may take you longer than 21 days to change this particular habit, especially if you have chosen one that is difficult to change.

STEP 6

Checkpoint no. 2 on day 14

You are in the second week of your transformation, and hopefully it is going as expected. If you are having success, you can offer yourself a new reward.

We encourage you to persevere.

If you have begun to skip days, it will be important to revisit the actions you identified to meet your goal. Identify the obstacles incurred and find new solutions.

Correspond with your coach. If you haven't chosen one, it may be a good idea to do so now.

STEP 7

After 21 days

MAINTAIN:

You have succeeded! You have completed the 21 days with your new habit and you have successfully kept the new habit during the 21 days. You can now enter the maintaining stage. Refer to the Prochaska model on the next page. At this stage, continue your efforts to make sure you keep the habit. A relapse is always possible, so beware!

If you are confident, you can decide to choose another habit to improve your well-being or you can take a break before taking on a new challenge.

RELAPSE:

- *Don't be discouraged!*
- *Pinpoint why you have failed.*
- *Find solutions to increase your chances of success.*
- *Create a new plan, talk to your coach for more support.*
- *Increase your motivation: remind yourself why you are making the change and the benefits you will reap.*

(An example for physical activity: Motivation to feel better, have more energy, lose weight, be stronger, get rid of back pain, have confidence, lead by example.)

! ATTENTION

It is likely that you will have to complete the 21-day process more than once, depending on your level of motivation and the difficulty of the habit change.

ARE YOU READY?

Know that to make changes in your lifestyle, you must be very motivated. You have to mentally prepare. For each habit, ask yourself the question: "Can I change this habit for the rest of my life?" If you answered no, obviously you will have a hard a time keeping your new habit.

You will find below a diagram of the Prochaska model, which demonstrates the steps of a behavioural change.

You have bought this book. You are probably at the stage of preparation or action. At least, we hope so! We wish you good luck in your process of lifestyle change. We encourage you during your journey. If you are still at a contemplative or pre-contemplative stage, read the steps calmly, take your time, and take inspiration from the medical information and statistics to motivate your change and to transition you into the preparation stage.

Don't get discouraged, no matter what obstacles or difficulties you face. If you don't succeed on the first try, try again. It is possible that certain habits will be harder to change than others.

GOOD LUCK!

Doctor James Prochaska wrote more than 300 publications on the dynamics of behavioural change to improve health and prevent disease.

He is the director of the Cancer Prevention Research Center, and a professor at the University of Rhode Island.

PROCHASKA
MODEL DIAGRAM

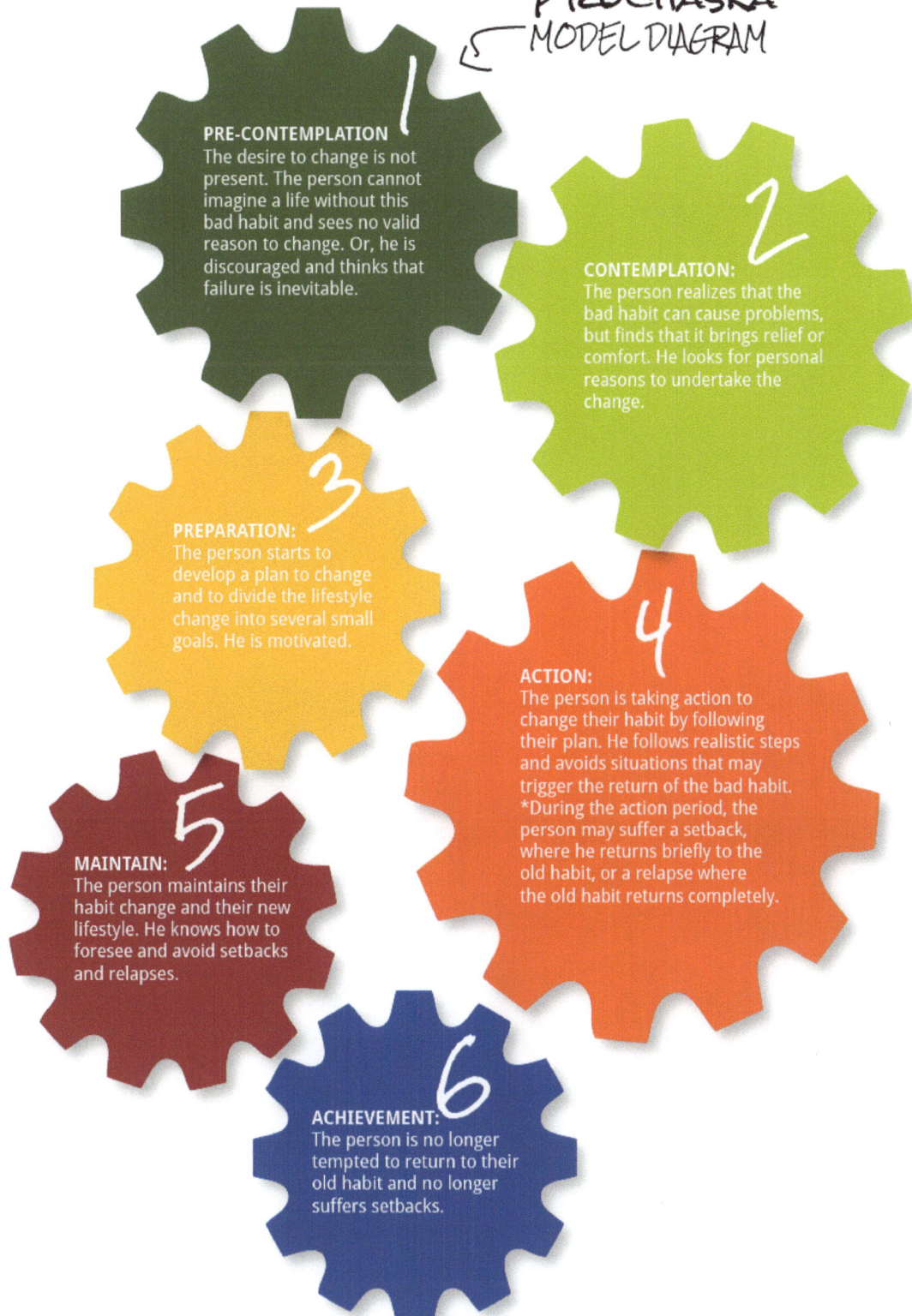

1

PRE-CONTEMPLATION
The desire to change is not present. The person cannot imagine a life without this bad habit and sees no valid reason to change. Or, he is discouraged and thinks that failure is inevitable.

2

CONTEMPLATION:
The person realizes that the bad habit can cause problems, but finds that it brings relief or comfort. He looks for personal reasons to undertake the change.

3

PREPARATION:
The person starts to develop a plan to change and to divide the lifestyle change into several small goals. He is motivated.

4

ACTION:
The person is taking action to change their habit by following their plan. He follows realistic steps and avoids situations that may trigger the return of the bad habit. *During the action period, the person may suffer a setback, where he returns briefly to the old habit, or a relapse where the old habit returns completely.

5

MAINTAIN:
The person maintains their habit change and their new lifestyle. He knows how to foresee and avoid setbacks and relapses.

6

ACHIEVEMENT:
The person is no longer tempted to return to their old habit and no longer suffers setbacks.

TO MOTIVATE YOU

While I was writing this book, I tried to undo a habit I've had for more than 40 years. A nervous tic, very difficult to control, started shortly after the passing of my mother. I remove the skin around my fingernails. As a result of my cuticle biting, a callous formed that has only made the bad habit worse, since I want to remove this hardened skin. I told myself that the publication of the guide would be a good motivation to free myself from this bad habit.

My motivation level was very high. I found that succeeding in this habit change would be a great example for the reader due to the high level of difficulty. Although, this type of habit is usually impossible to get rid of. Therefore, I filled in the 21-day logbook and determined all the actions I would need to take to stop this bad habit.

In 40 years, I had already tried many, many times without success. While applying this method, I had to complete several 21-day cycles. I can also testify that I am still at the Maintain/Relapse stage, but I refuse to give up.

I encourage you, then, to persevere, no matter how hard the desired change.

I can assure you that the results will make it worthwhile.

After all the consultations I offered, people that made lifestyle changes were very satisfied afterwards. They could not have imagined what their life would have been like without these changes. The satisfaction and well being achieved felt worthwhile.

Don't wait...

Change your lifestyle and you will see the results!

Isabelle Lipari

SECTION 1

NUTRITION

1. Drink more water
2. Eat more fruits
3. Eat more vegetables
4. Eliminate soft drinks
5. Choose healthy snacks
6. Eat a proper breakfast
7. Eat less junk food
8. Eat less red meat
9. Eat more fish
10. Avoid snacks after dinner
11. Achieve energy balance
12. Eliminate French fries
13. Drink less coffee

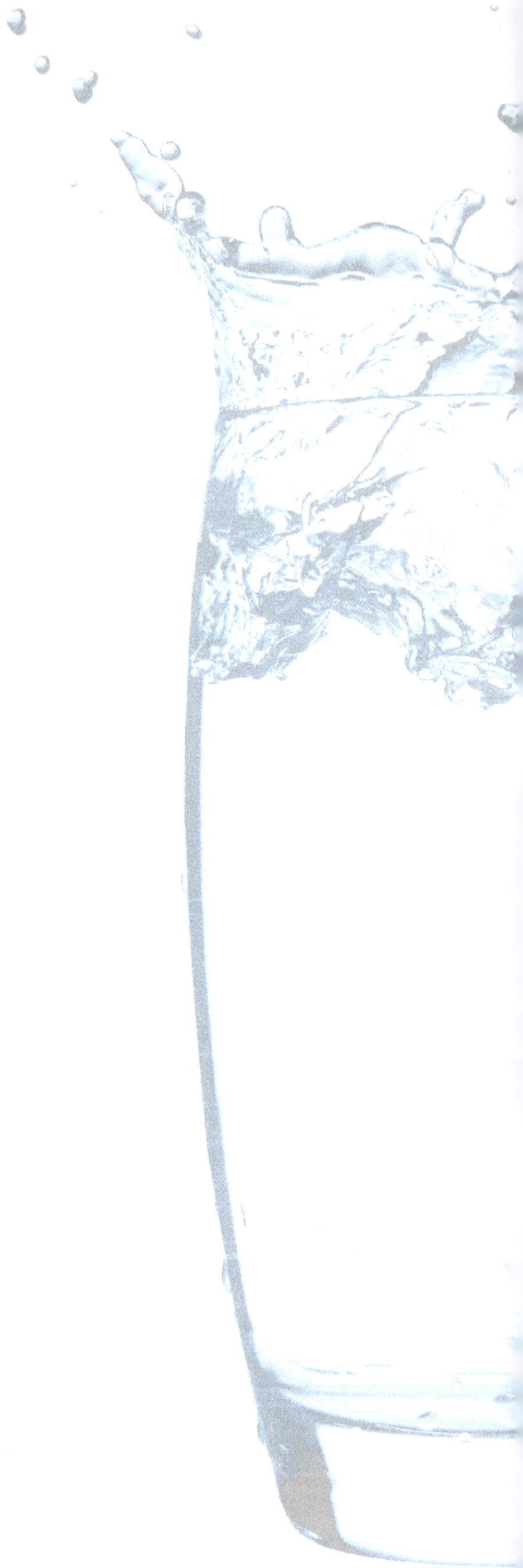

HABIT 1
DRINK MORE WATER

Water is one of life's indispensable resources. Our cells are made up of 70-95% water. Man cannot survive more than one week without water since water is responsible for a variety of vital chemical processes. The fatigue felt at the end of a day is often attributed to dehydration. Furthermore, by the time we are thirsty, it is often too late and our body is already dehydrated.

Sadly, we never learned to drink water daily. As children, we were given juice, milk, or worse, soft drinks. Most of us don't drink enough water to hydrate and to ensure that our body functions properly.

☞ GOAL

Drink at least 8 ounces (250 ml) of water twice a day, on top of other sources of liquid over the course of the day: soup, fruits and vegetables containing a lot of water (celery, melon, cucumber...).

HOW?

1 Get a reusable 8 or 16-ounce (250 or 500 ml) water bottle. There are many now that are insulated or that have a spill-proof cap, like the CamelBak or Contigo. Beware of plastics that contain BPA. Nalgene bottles do not. If you do not want to use a bottle, make sure to keep a glass of water at arms reach.

2 Fill your bottle or glass every morning. Drink at least 16 ounces (500 ml) each day.

3 Make sure to always have it with you, no matter where you go.

4 Try to drink throughout the day; water instead of juice, soft drinks, and energy drinks.

HEALTH INFO

Thirst is without a doubt the way the human body tells us it is in a state of dehydration. Eventually, this proves detrimental to the proper functioning of the body.

In general, an adult of average size, living in a temperate region and not engaging in much physical activity, needs around 2.5 litres a day with around 1 litre coming from food and 1.5 litres from liquids.

Bisphenol A (BPA) is an industrial chemical found in polycarbonate, a clear and hard type of plastic. Recycling codes numbers 1 through 6 are not made of polycarbonate therefore do not contain BPA. Recycling code number 7 however, represents all other types of plastics including polycarbonate. Plastics with this code may or may not contain BPA, although it is often indicated on products if they are BPA free.

HOW?

1 Eat fruits in the morning with breakfast or in a smoothie (frozen fruit).

2 As a snack, around 10:30 AM.

3 As a snack, around 3:00 PM.

4 Incorporate it into your meals with salads, sandwiches, or meats. Here are some suggestions:

Grapes, apples, oranges, mandarins, pears or any kind of dried fruit in salads; green or red apple slices, sliced pears in sandwiches with chicken, ham, brie or any cheese; pork fillet with apples/plums/grapes, chicken or tofu with pineapple, pork roast with grapefruit.

5 Bring enough for the week to work every Monday morning, and if possible, a little basket for your workstation. Having fruit nearby will help to remind you to eat them, and will create the habit to do so.

HABIT 2
EAT MORE FRUITS

Canada's Food Guide recommends that women between the ages of 19 and 50 consume 7 or 8 servings of fruits and vegetables a day, and that men should consume between 8 and 10. Vegetables are better for you than fruits, the latter containing natural sugar, therefore more c

☞ GOAL

Consume between 3 and 4 servings of fruits a day.

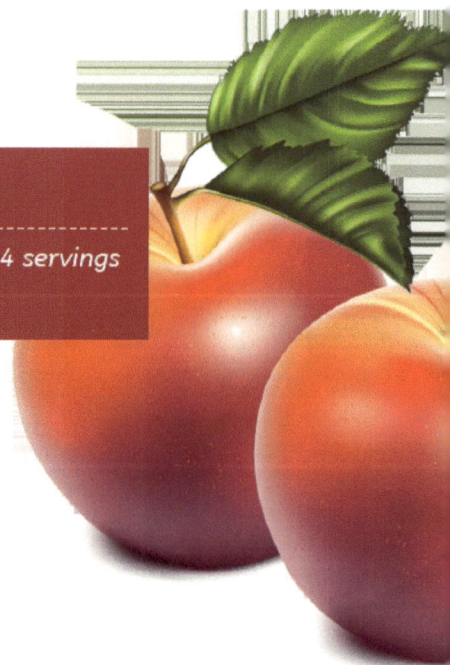

⚕ HEALTH INFO

Fruits and vegetables (mainly vegetables) contain few calories, but a lot of water. Pick up the habit of eating a good amount. Fill your plate! On top of providing vitamins and minerals, fruits and vegetables help to maintain a healthy weight.

According to the Government of Canada, a diet rich with fruits and vegetables can contribute to reducing the risk of certain types of cancer and can also reduce the risk of heart disease.

For more information on the nutrient intake of fruits and vegetables, consult appendix 5 to 8.

HOW?

1   Always carry a good serving of raw vegetables in your lunch box if you bring your lunch to work. If you often eat out, choose salads or sandwiches that contain grilled vegetables or a sandwich with a choice of one or two salads. Beware of mayonnaise-based dressing; they contain more calories.

2   Afternoon snack: Mixed vegetables, hummus, soy dip, vegetable drink.

3   Choose a vegetable juice with a meal or snack (a 156 ml can contains the equivalent of one serving of vegetables). Be careful of the salt content for those who are hypertensive, favour the reduced-sodium version.

4   Dinner: Always include at least two vegetable servings and a salad. Lessen the meat portion to make room for the vegetables. In general, we have a tendency to fill our plates with a large serving of meat, leaving little room for vegetables.

HABIT 3

EAT MORE VEGETABLES

3

According to the Government of Canada's recommendation, the ideal intake is 4 to 6 vegetable servings a day.

Fruits and vegetables are excellent foods:

- High in fibre
- High in water
- High in vitamins and minerals
- High in antioxidants
- Low in calories

⌖ GOAL

Consume between 4 and 6 servings of vegetables a day.

Here are some other meal suggestions that incorporate vegetable servings into your daily diet:

Salad as a meal at lunch or even at dinner. Salads should not be reserved for the hot season only. They are delicious all the time.

Homemade soup: Add all the vegetables that you have on hand. When cooking in the broth, all their nutrients are retained in the soup.

HABIT 4
ELIMINATE SOFT DRINKS

This bad habit is very difficult to change. The number of people that consume large quantities of soft drinks every day, with little regard for the health effects, is astounding. Even more shocking is that many parents give them to their children as young as two years old! Many people keep soft drinks in the house at all times, "just in case." As a result, they are always readily available for the family. Realistically, soft drinks should be reserved for parties, family events, or other special events.

☑ GOAL

Reduce or eliminate the consumption of soft drinks.

HOW?

1 First, evaluate your current consumption. One option is to cut your consumption gradually instead of stopping completely. For example, if you drink soft drinks every day of the week, you can choose to cut one day out completely, or you can cut down your daily consumption.

2 Record your current daily consumption.

3 Write down a final consumption goal.

4 Choose a reduction method, daily or weekly.

5 Find a replacement, ideally water; a coffee or tea in moderate quantity is also acceptable.

To motivate yourself, it is good to remember that soft drinks are full of sugar and the "diet" versions are filled with chemical sweetener. Neither is good for you.

19kg!

The amount of sugar ingested per year if you drink one 355 ml can each day

see also:
www.youtube.com/
watch?v=UndXrdEY2MI

HEALTH INFO

Soft drinks contain no nutritional value. Not only do they contain a large quantity of sugar (9 teaspoons), regular consumption of these beverages has numerous harmful consequences to the health of individuals. For example, obesity, type 2 diabetes, cardiovascular diseases, dental health, bone health, certain types of cancer, kidney stones.

CHOOSE HEALTHY SNACKS

5

HOW?

1 Decide if you want to add a snack to your routine or change the choice of snack.

2 Choose snacks such as: fresh fruits, raw vegetables, hard or cottage cheeses, whole wheat crackers, nuts and dried fruits or trail mix, yogurt (with or without granola), etc.

3 Avoid at all costs snacks rich in trans fats in the afternoon. They are difficult to digest and you will find yourself getting sleepy. Also, they are unhealthy (chips, potato chips, soft drinks, chocolate bars, candies and other treats often found in vending machines).

4 Keep healthy choices around at all times, it will help. If you have access to a refrigerator at work, great! Take advantage by bringing enough for the week! You can store fruits (keep a basket at work), nuts or mixtures of nuts in an airtight container. Each day, you should bring only perishable goods (dairy products, raw veggies and other foods).

Eating a snack in the morning and in the afternoon is strongly recommended. More and more studies show that eating 5 to 6 small meals a day help to maintain a healthy weight. Firstly, you will find yourself less hungry between meals. It will also help you accumulate the 7 to 10 servings of fruits and vegetables you need. Then, you will be energized by the healthy foods and your days will be more productive. By consequence, you will be prompted to continue eating fruits and vegetables and less junk food – every day.

GOAL

Eat two snacks per day.

HEALTH INFO

Maintaining a balance of energy all day long by eating more small meals helps to reduce the problems of slow metabolism, maintain muscle mass and reach the total daily nutrients the body needs.

EAT A NUTRITIOUS BREAKFAST

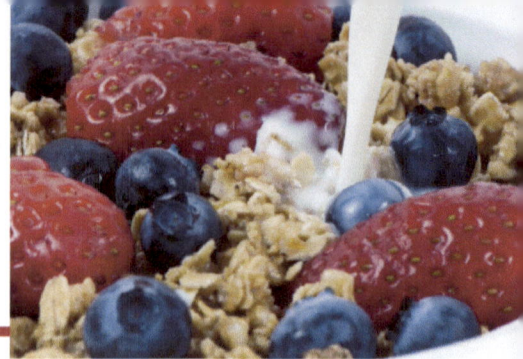

Breakfast is to our bodies what gasoline is to a car. Many people skip breakfast completely, which is very bad for your long-term health. You will find yourself feeling empty; your body goes into survival mode and will start using its energy stores. You will be lacking the energy to function both physically and mentally.

⌖ GOAL

Eat a proper breakfast every morning.

HOW?

1 A good breakfast consists of the following: Carbohydrates, proteins, fruits. Choose what pleases you the most: Roasted grains, cereal, oatmeal, eggs, yogurt and granola, fruit or vegetable smoothie, granola bar, etc.

2 Wake up just 5 minutes earlier if you find that you never have enough time. Make your breakfast while you get ready, or eat while you get ready. You can also find something to eat on the go: a smoothie, a granola bar or simply a fruit like an apple or banana.

3 You can choose to start this habit with a liquid breakfast or by eating once you get to work, if you find it difficult to eat solid foods early in the morning.

4 Start with small amounts.

5 Build a regular routine to include this meal daily.

6 You can prepare certain things the night before, preparing the coffee, setting the table and getting the food ready for the morning.

⚕ HEALTH INFO

At a neuroscience conference in 2012, a study showed that subjects who didn't eat breakfast consumed 20 calories more over the course of the day than the subjects that ate a good breakfast.

EAT LESS JUNK FOOD

Eliminating junk food from our diet seems impossible for some. But fear not, it is possible! The less you eat it, the less your body craves it. You will find that when you do make an exception, your body will have a tough time digesting it. The trans fats found in most junk foods are extremely unhealthy. They are responsible for many current diseases. (See the table on trans fats in appendix 13).

⌖ GOAL

Decrease junk food intake.

HOW?

1 Take a look at your current habits. What are the situations where you find yourself choosing to eat junk food instead of a good meal? Is it lack of time? Influence from colleagues or friends? Accessibility? Your schedule? Lack of planning?

2 Once you have determined the situations in which you eat junk food, figure out the change you would like to make. For example, if you notice you're eating too much junk at work, bring your lunch instead or choose healthier restaurants.

3 Reduce slowly. This way is easier and more likely to produce long-term success. Eliminate one fast food meal per week and replace it with a home cooked meal or a healthy choice of restaurant. There are more and more food options that are fast AND healthy.

4 Plan your meals, for lunch and dinner. Planning will help you keep the ingredients around in order to cook healthy meals. This will stop you from eating on the go because of lack of time (see habit 22).

5 Carry healthy snacks. If your junk habits derive from poor choices and eating out of vending machines, you have to make better choices or ban yourself from vending machines!

6 Choose good fats like olive oils, canola, and grape seed. Our body needs fats; we shouldn't deprive it. It is possible you have become addicted to trans fats, which are often present in packaged foods. This will be difficult to undo.

7 Save fast food or junk food (treats, chips, sweets, etc.) for exceptional or special circumstances: once a week, or better, once a month.

HEALTH INFO

" *Every year in France, junk food causes three times as many deaths as tobacco and fifty times as many as car accidents. It is in part responsible for 30% of cancer cases, 500 000 heart failures cases, 2 million cases of diabetes, and 8 million cases of obesity.*"

Le point, France, 2009

HABIT 8
EAT LESS RED MEAT

Our education and our traditions have accustomed us to eat a lot of meat, mainly red meat. Our meals consist often of one big serving and it has become difficult to even imagine a meal without including meat of some sort.

With age, red meat becomes harmful for many people, especially those with cardiovascular diseases, high blood pressure, high cholesterol or heart problems. In these cases, doctors will recommend eating less red meat.

However, proteins perform several vital functions in our body. So make sure to consume enough and replace meat with equivalent sources.

Here are some substitutes:

• Legumes, nuts and whole grains.
• Eggs
• Tofu and soy products
• Chicken
• Fish and shellfish

HOW?

1 Evaluate your current weekly amount of red meat.

2 State a goal to reduce it.

3 Identify some substitutes from the list below.

4 Find interesting recipes with those choices.

5 Plan the week's menu, which will ensure you have enough substitute products and avoid falling to the easiest solutions (see habit 22).

⌖ GOAL

Consume a maximum of 3 servings of red meat per week.

HEALTH INFO

Many scientific studies show more and more that there is a link between the consumption of red meat and colon cancer. In effect, consuming only 100g of red meat a day would increase the risk by 29%.

An increase of the risks of cancer of the oesophagus, pancreas, lungs, stomach, endometrium, and prostate would also be identified. Processed meats (50g of cold meats or deli per day) – increases the risk by 20%. Heavy consumption of red meat can also cause obesity, another important risk factor of cancer.

The Canadian Cancer Society recommends an even smaller amount with a maximum of 300g per week, 3 servings of 85g to 100g (3oz), which is about the size of a deck of cards!

HABIT 9
EAT MORE FISH

The North American population does not eat enough fish. The Japanese and Mediterranean eat a lot of it, and consequently benefit from better health and live longer. On Okinawa Island, where the habitants' diet is rich in fish and vegetables, there are 3 to 5 times more centenarians than in France.

Mediterranean people also have a rich diet of fish, and generally have better cardiovascular health. Several studies show that this diet can prevent cardiovascular diseases, cancer, type 2 diabetes, Alzheimer's, and brain aging.

⌖ GOAL

Eat at least two servings of fish per week.

HOW?

1   If, like many people, you don't like fish, try to include it at least once a week to start.

2   Start with fish such as salmon and trout. They are the best tasting and the least "rubbery."

3   Serve them with healthy seasonings (tamari, garlic, olive oil, capers, onions, lemons, spices).

4   Once you are used to it and have acquired the taste, you can try other types of fish from your grocery store or favourite fishmonger.

9

HEALTH INFO

According to a study published in the Journal of the American Medical Association, eating fish once or twice a week reduces the likelihood of death caused by a coronary heart disease by 36%, and deaths from all causes by 17%.

The consumption of fish, and in particular the Omega-3 fatty acids they contain, will have health benefits such as the reduction of cardiovascular disease. All fish, but in particular "fatty fish" like salmon, mackerel, trout, and sardines, contain significant amounts of Omega-3 fatty acids, making them beneficial for your health.

Fish is also an excellent source of protein, calcium, and minerals (like phosphorous, iron, selenium, and potassium) and certain vitamins (like thiamine, riboflavin, and niacin), all the important elements for the maintenance of optimal health.

HOW?

1 Keep track of the time and foods you tend to eat at night.

2 Write down your reason(s) for this urge (for example, boredom, sadness, anxiety, hunger, fatigue, lack of energy, or by habit).

3 Write down what you do while you eat your snack.

4 Convince yourself that you do not absolutely need to eat at night.

5 Change the habits that surround this moment of hunger. If you are in front of the computer when you feel the desire to eat, do something else for the first few days. Phone a friend for example, or take a walk, etc.

6 Replace your snack with a glass of water, a cup of tea or herbal tea.

7 If you have difficulty eliminating this bad habit, opt for lower-calorie, healthier snacks (see suggestions).

HABIT 10
AVOID SNACKS AFTER DINNER

Studies do not prove that eating before bedtime actually causes weight gain. It is actually the nature of the foods you eat as well as the total number of calories eaten in the day that are the most harmful. Most people who eat at night are eating sweets or salty/fatty foods while sitting in front of the television or another screen.

Another problem would be the acid created in the stomach by eating snacks close to bedtime. Furthermore, certain foods interfere with sleep.

If your desire to eat at night is uncontrollable or you wish to reduce your total overall caloric intake, it will be preferable to change the foods you eat.

⌖ GOAL

Eliminate snacks after dinner or choose something healthier.

HEALTH INFO

Research from Harvard Medical School does not endorse the theory that eating before bedtime causes weight gain. In fact, the entirety of calories ingested during the day has a greater impact on weight as well as the type of foods you eat at night (that are often sugary or salty treats).

Here are the best and healthiest choices that actually induce sleep:

- *Cherries*
- *A glass of water*
- *Yogurt, with or without granola*
- *Whole grain cereal*
- *A banana*
- *Chamomile or herbal tea*

HABIT 11
ACHIEVE ENERGY BALANCE

How many people eat too much relative to their energy requirement? Almost everyone.

Indeed, we pick up bad habits as children and in our twenties – habits that our bodies can no longer sustain in our thirties. Here are some examples:

- Eating a fourth meal in the middle of the night.
- Eating two dinners instead of just one.
- Eating junk food too often or as a snack.
- Eating before bed
- Eating dessert after every meal.

Men especially are taken with this bad habit because their caloric demand during growth is very high. They eat a lot, but do not reduce the quantities they eat as they mature. Women, on the other hand, tend to pick up this bad habit during pregnancy or breastfeeding. Women's nutritional needs during this period are much higher, so they consume more, rightfully so. But once the baby arrives or breastfeeding is finished, they should return to their original eating habits.

HOW?

1 Put a little less food on your plate for each meal, until you have achieved a reasonable portion*. In reducing your portions slowly, the size of your stomach will slowly shrink.

*A reasonable portion: you should be able to see the bottom of the plate; the food shouldn't form a mountain. There should be more vegetables than proteins or carbs.

2 If hunger strikes, eat low-calorie foods, like raw vegetables or hard cheeses, or even fruits, a small amount of nuts or yogurt.

3 Eat more (5 or 6) smaller meals rather than 2 or 3 large ones. Listen to your body and stop eating once you are full.

4 Eat more slowly so you don't overeat. Your brain will get the signal that you are full.

11

⌖ GOAL

Reduce the number of calories according to personal goals. (See appendix 9 – Weight loss)

HEALTH INFO

The majority of women and elderly need 1600 calories a day. Kids, young girls, active women and most men need around 2200 calories. Young boys and active men need 2800 calories a day.

CALORIE REQUIREMENTS – MEN

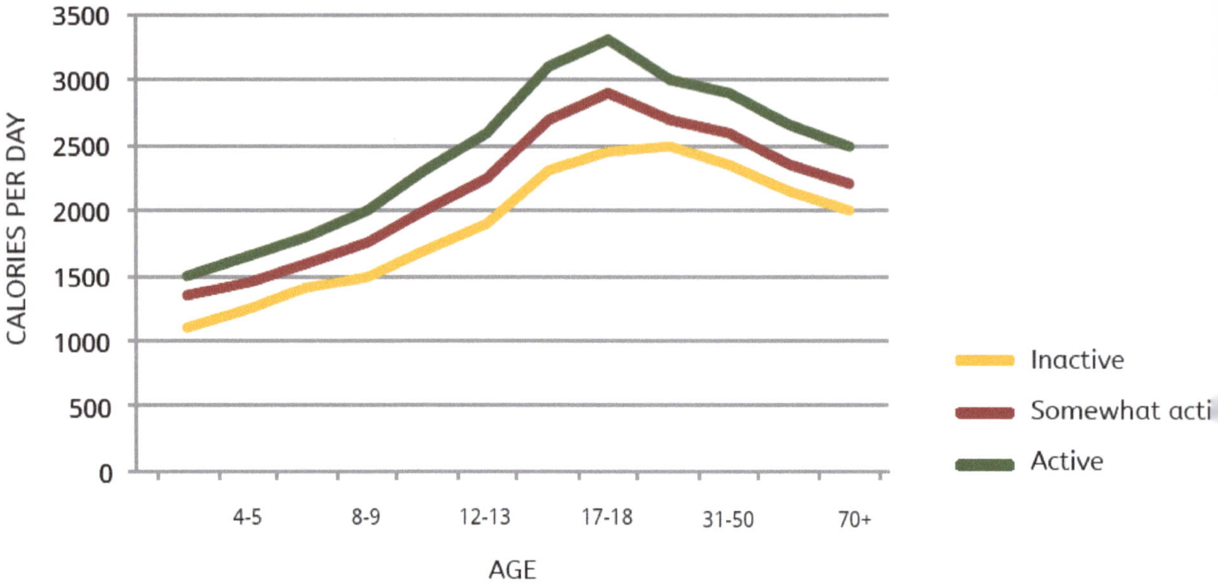
3500
3000
2500
2000
1500
1000
500
0
CALORIES PER DAY
4-5
8-9
12-13
17-18
31-50
70+
AGE
Inactive
Somewhat acti
Active

CALORIE REQUIREMENTS – WOMEN

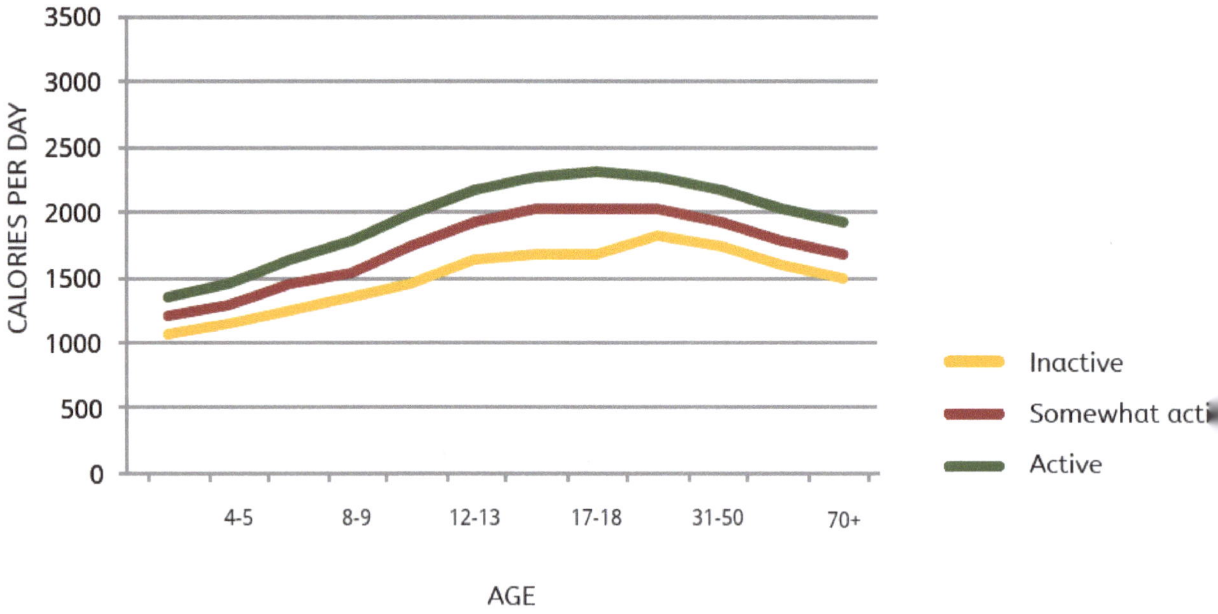
3500
3000
2500
2000
1500
1000
500
0
CALORIES PER DAY
4-5
8-9
12-13
17-18
31-50
70+
AGE
Inactive
Somewhat acti
Active

HABIT 12
ELIMINATE FRENCH FRIES

Fries are so good! But only once in a while...

Resisting the temptation to order fries in a restaurant is hard. Especially if you are eating in a restaurant every day and they offer you fries on the side.

Fries are filled with trans fats and calories. Not only are they bad for your cardiovascular health, but they are also full of empty calories. Beware of how many you eat; it can add up quickly on the scale.

1 Keep track of how many servings you consume this week.

2 Reduce this quantity gradually. For example, if you eat fries every day, it would be very difficult to immediately reduce to once a month (ideal goal). You will probably want to try two servings a week at first, then once a week.

3 To start, choose a quantity that you can achieve, that you can attain without getting discouraged.

4 Identify the ways to help you stay on track. For example, avoid restaurants, choose those that don't serve fries, reduce portions (opt for half fries, half salad) etc.

12

⚙ GOAL
Eat fries only once a month.

HEALTH INFO

According to various sources and depending on the size, a poutine can reach between 710 and 950 calories in a small or regular size, standard recipe of three main ingredients. After eating one, you would have to do between two and three hours of moderate cardiovascular activity (running, elliptical, biking, or other) to burn it off! For a regular serving of fries, figure about 270 calories and just under an hour of cardio.

TYPE OF EXERCISE

CALORIES BURNED
PER HOUR BY WEIGHT

	130lbs./59kg	155 lbs./68kg	180 lbs./82kg	205 lbs./93kg
Shovelling snow	354	422	490	558
Downhill skiing	295	352	409	465
Soccer	413	493	572	651
Squash	708	844	981	1117
Moderate stationary bike	413	493	572	651
Stretching and yoga	236	281	327	372
Swimming	413	493	572	651
Tennis	413	493	572	651
Martial arts	590	704	817	931
Jogging	472	563	654	745
Speed walking	224	267	311	354
Low-intensity bodybuilding	177	211	245	279
High-intensity bodybuilding	354	422	490	558
Biking on moderate route	472	563	654	745
Aerobics	384	457	531	605
Badmington	266	317	368	419
Golf + carrying bag	266	317	368	419
Golf + pulling bag	254	303	351	400
Golf + cart	207	246	286	326
Cross-country skiing	472	563	654	745
Gardening	236	281	327	372
General housework	207	246	286	326

1 Evaluate your coffee consumption over a week period. Identify the moments in the day when you have some.

2 Establish the number of coffees you need to cut out. Depending on your habits, it is preferable to reduce slowly rather than suddenly. The significant, sudden decrease of caffeine in your body can prove to be difficult to adjust to and can cause headaches.

3 Find a drink to replace coffee. Water is the best option (see habit 1) or even green tea. Beware of teas; some of them have just as much caffeine as coffee. Green tea contains many health benefits, therefore it is a healthy choice. A healthy snack can help give you the energy you were getting from caffeine.

HABIT 13
DRINK LESS COFFEE

Despite the fact that coffee is a natural product, it becomes toxic in strong doses, since caffeine has harmful effects on the human body. The acceptable quantity of coffee per day is 3 to 4 cups (clearly, these are coffees of normal size, an 8 ounce/250ml cup, and not the enlarged sizes sold in cafés).

The problem often starts at work, where people drink coffee like we're supposed to drink water, in other words, several times a day, as a habit, out of boredom or to boost their energy level.

Too much caffeine every day can cause palpitations, headaches, stomach aches, insomnia, tremors and tachycardia, among other things. In reasonable doses, coffee is a good source of antioxidants, keeps the brain stimulated and prevents certain illnesses like Parkinson's or Alzheimer's (demonstrated experimentally but still under review).

13

☉ GOAL

Reduce coffee intake to around 3 cups of 120 to 250 ml (6 to 8 ounces) a day.

⚕ HEALTH INFO

Coffee can be beneficial in moderate quantities (200-300mg a day), according to several studies on the subject. This represents about two or three cups of filtered coffee. At equal amount, espresso coffees contain less caffeine than filtered coffee.

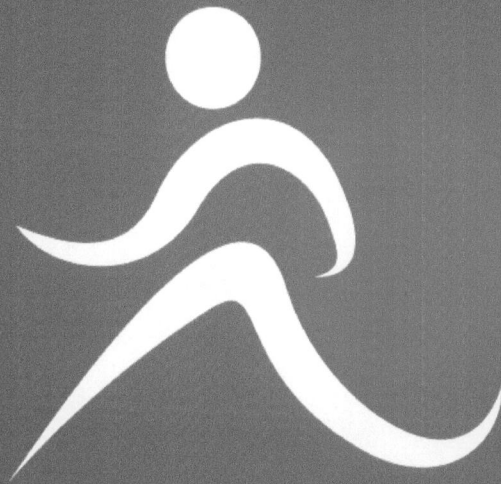

SECTION 2

PHYSICAL ACTIVITY

14. Become active

15. Start walking

16. Improve flexibility

17. Integrate exercise into your daily routine

18. Be active, even at work

19. Start an intensive workout

This section covers daily physical activities, performed at different levels of intensity. Exercise brings benefits to your health and wellness, stress management, mood, and energy level. Listed below are all the advantages to engaging in physical activity, advantages that also apply to all the habits presented in this section.

THE BENEFITS OF ENGAGING IN PHYSICAL ACTIVITY:

Reduces the risk of premature death

Reduces the risk of cardiovascular disease

Decreases the resting heart rate

Helps maintain normal blood pressure

Improves the efficiency of the heart

Increases muscle mass and decrease body fat

Increases HDL cholesterol (good cholesterol) and reduce LDL (bad cholesterol)

Reduces the risk of developing Type 2 diabetes

Promotes joint stability

Increases muscular strength

Strengthens bones

Increases the rate of metabolism

Improves core strength and stability

Improves the strength of back muscles

Improves balance, coordination and agility

Improves body image and confidence

Reduces the risk of depression and anxiety

Helps manage stress

When we begin doing a physical activity, the amount of oxygen circulating through our body increases, as soon as our breathing increases. The brain then releases endorphins, the famous happy hormones. These hormones help to increase our sense of well-being, like during moments when laughter overtakes us or intense moments of joy.

WARNING

Before undergoing any physical activity, fill out the "Physical Activity Readiness Questionnaire (PAR-Q)" in appendix 10, to clearly identify if you have any special conditions preventing you from exercising. This form will determine whether you should consult your doctor before making the physical changes you wish to achieve.

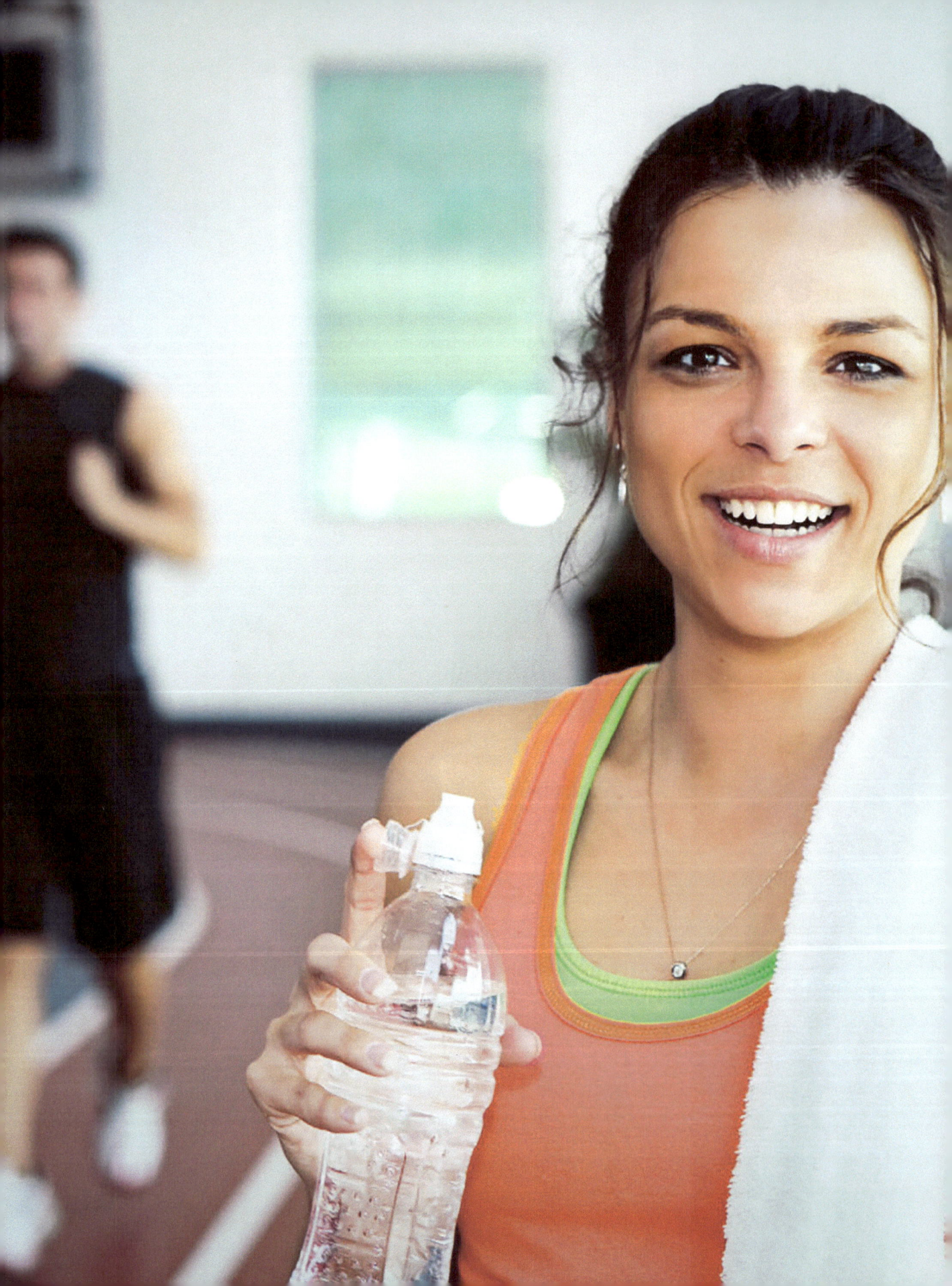

1 Always park your car a little further from your destination.

2 Take the stairs instead of the elevator, start with a few floors at a time.

3 Get up to go see a colleague instead of sending an email.

4 Speak on the phone standing up instead of sitting.

5 Ride a bike or walk to travel short distances.

6 Do some stretching and exercises during the day at your desk.

7 When in a standing position (for example, in line), practice good posture:
- Stand up very straight
- Tilt the pelvis forward
- Extend your torso and spine
- Contract the gluteal and abdominal muscles

8 When in a seated position, contract the gluteal and abdominal muscles and keep the back straight. Repeat these muscular contractions several times.

HABIT 14
BECOME ACTIVE

You are totally inactive and you would like to incorporate some physical activity into your routine without devoting too much time. This might be the case of parents with young children, those with parents to take care of, or with a loved one that is ill. Despite the lack of time, it is important to move and stay active. All forms of physical activity count!

14

⌖ GOAL

Incorporate physical activities into daily tasks.

HEALTH INFO

According to the World Health Organization, inactivity doubles the risks of cardiovascular diseases, diabetes, and obesity, and increases the risks of colon cancer, hypertension, osteoporosis, lipid disorders, depression and anxiety.

HABIT 15
START WALKING

Walking is a simple, accessible, and easy physical activity that can be done at any time. In addition to its physical benefits, it can allow you to free your mind, enjoy the landscape and reduce stress levels.

⚐ GOAL

Take a five-minute walk every day.

You probably think that 5 minutes is too short and insufficient a time to start getting healthy. Start with 5 minutes, this short period can easily fit in your schedule.

Develop the habit of doing some physical activity every day; it will bring you satisfaction and encouragement. Five minutes is better than nothing at all! Also, the five minute walk will easily turn into 10 or 15.

HOW?

1 Choose the time best suited to your schedule.

2 Write it in your agenda like an appointment, either in the morning or after a meal.

3 Get a good pair of walking shoes. It could be a running shoe or a good walking shoe. In winter, you will need winter boots or hiking boots.

4 While walking, practice deep breathing (see habit 20). Breathe in through the nose and breathe out through the mouth. Adapt your breathing rhythm to your walking speed.

5 Make sure to keep a moderate to fast pace in order to achieve benefits.

6 Try to clear your mind and only think of your breathing and your visual field.

✠ HEALTH INFO

Walking is beneficial toward the body's maintenance of flexible and nimble joints. It develops muscle tone especially since the repeated arm movement simultaneously relaxes the upper body. The heart's health will be improved as well, since it is also a muscle – do not forget that! Walking is also an effective way to lose or maintain weight if it is done on a regular basis.

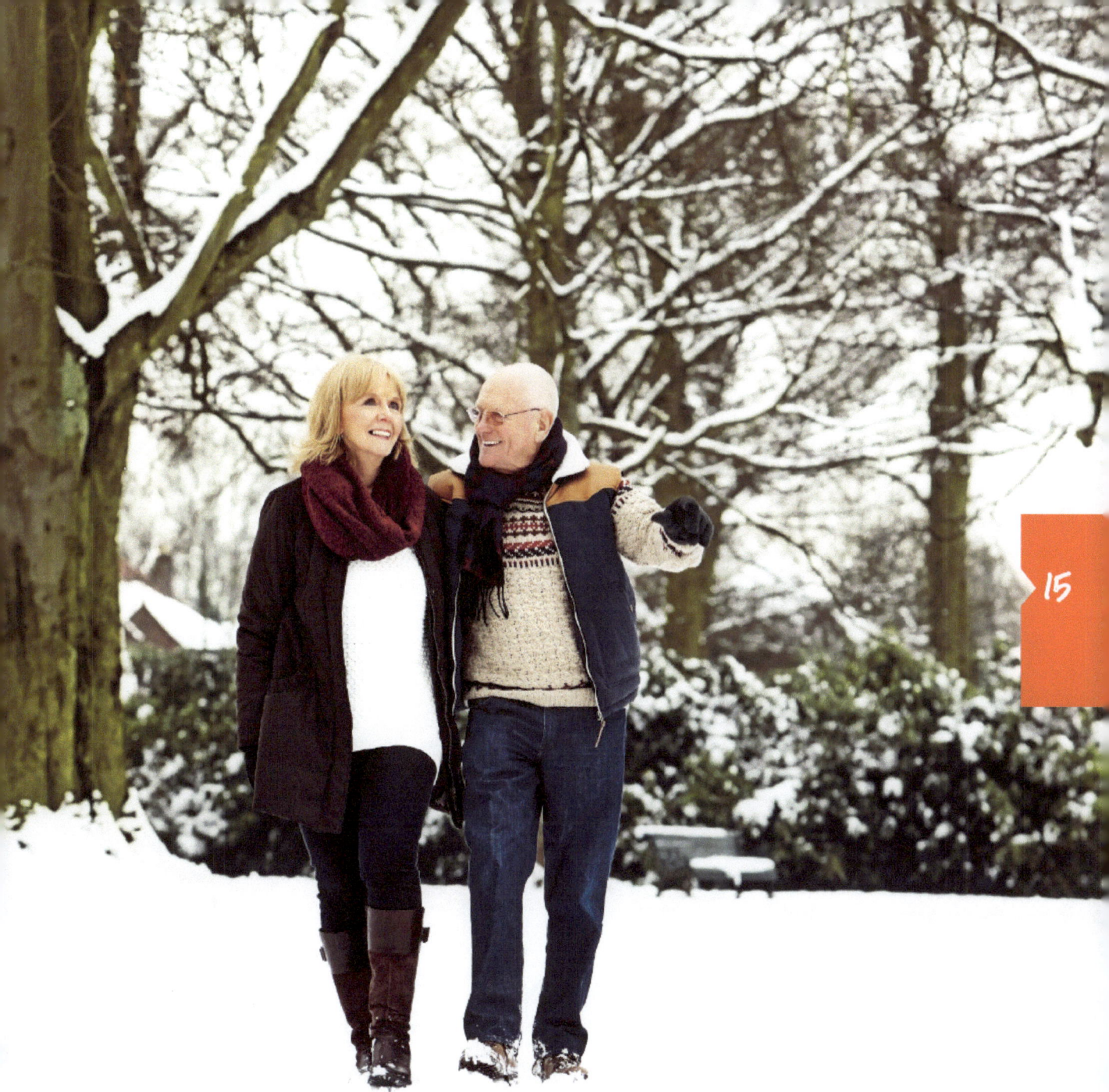

INCREASE THE LENGTH OF YOUR WALKS

You've now walked 5 minutes, every day for 21 days. You have completed your first cycle. Congratulations! Now you have decided to walk for a longer period of time.

1. Walk at a good pace and don't forget to maintain deep abdominal breathing throughout.
2. Make sure to record the walk in your agenda. You can also invite a co-worker or a friend.
3. Continue until you have walked at a good pace for 10, 20 or 30 minutes.
4. Try reaching 30 minutes 3 to 4 times a week.

HABIT 16
IMPROVE YOUR FLEXIBILITY

If you are very inactive and the idea of a 5-minute walk makes you cringe, perhaps a stretching routine is the solution for you. Or perhaps you have noticed over time that you have lost some flexibility or are beginning to have joint pain. This program was designed for beginners and can be complete in less than 15 minutes. The stretches are excellent for those who are inactive and that don't move very much during the workday. The stretches are also quite relaxing.

HOW?

1 Print the stretching program (see appendix 11 for the stretching program).

2 Mark off a time in your calendar for stretching: when you wake up, at work when you are tense, or even before going to bed at night.

3 You can do the routine while listening to calming meditation or yoga music.

⌖ GOAL

Stretch 5 to 15 minutes a day, every day.

HEALTH INFO

Regularly doing flexibility exercises brings benefits such as muscle tone, blood circulation, stress management, and concentration. In addition, stretches help with mental and physical relaxation, improve the range of motion of joints, and help to prevent sore muscles, joint pain, and injury.

1 Before beginning, we remind you to fill out the PAR-Q in appendix 10.

2 Choose one or two of the activities you like.

3 Mark off the 30-minute time slots each day in your agenda. Keep in mind that you can also do several sessions of 10 or 15 minutes.

4 Make sure to have all the necessary equipment to do the chosen activity (good shoes or boots, sport equipment or other...).

5 Remember to start slowly to avoid injuries.

HABIT 17

INTEGRATE PHYSICAL ACTIVITY INTO YOUR DAILY ROUTINE

Health Canada recommends a minimum of 30 minutes of moderate physical activity a day. In 2011, the government reduced the number to 15 minutes so that the goal could be more attainable and more Canadians could reach the minimum. Nonetheless, try to reach 30 minutes a day; it is not that difficult.

It is also important to consider that some days we do more, and other days we do less. Concentrate on adding physical activity to your daily routine, just like taking a shower, eating, and brushing your teeth. That way, you will be more inclined to keep the habit without skipping days.

17

⌖ GOAL

Do 30 minutes of physical activity 4 or 5 days a week.

INDOOR ACTIVITIES

Walking or running on a treadmill

Stationary bike

Fitness classes in a private or group setting – dance, yoga, Zumba®, martial arts.

Physical training or conditioning in a private or group setting, including cardio, bodybuilding, and stretching

Swimming

Tennis

Team sports (Hockey, volleyball, basketball)

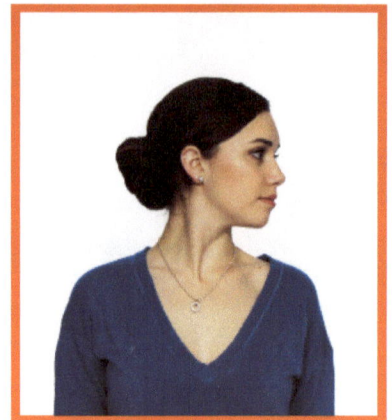

OUTDOOR ACTIVITIES

Walking or running (with winter boots or hiking boots for winter)

Cycling

Hiking

Swimming

Tennis

Cross country skiing

Snowshoeing

Various outdoor team sports

Skating

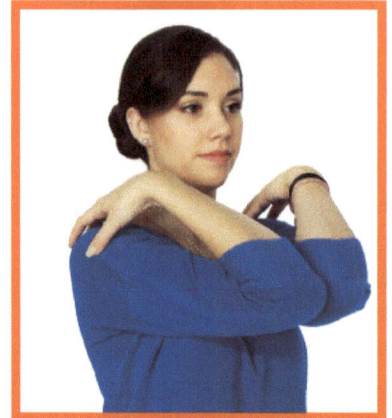

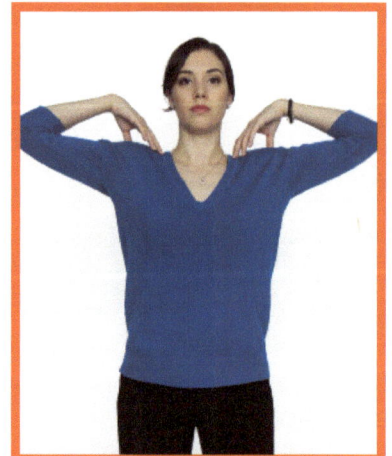

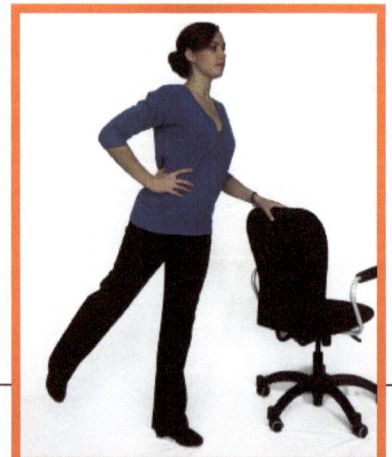

HABIT 18

BE ACTIVE, EVEN AT WORK

If you work in an office or in an environment where you have the opportunity to take a break, you can make a habit of doing exercises and stretches during the day, at your workstation or designated area.

1 Print appendix 12: 10-minute workout.

2 Establish your goal depending on your workload and what suits you best. Remember, it is always easier to change a habit slowly. Establish a realistic goal, do not get discouraged if you miss one or two sessions, and above all, persevere.

3 Record your exercise breaks in your agenda each day. It might help to program a timer on your computer. You may choose to do one of these programs:

a. 3 times a week, Mondays, Wednesdays and Fridays.

b. 4 times: Mondays, Tuesdays, Thursdays, Fridays.

c. All 5 days of the week (ideal).

d. The schedule of your choosing.

4 Complete the 10 minutes of strengthening/stretching over the course of the morning.

5 Complete the series in the afternoon.

6 Take a 10-minute walk at lunch or in the evening.

18

⌖ GOAL

Reach the 30 minutes of recommended physical activity over the course of a workday.

HEALTH INFO

According to a study by The Lancet Journal, men and women who are seated more than six hours a day diminish their life expectancy by 18% and 37% respectively. In effect, the damages caused by a prolonged seated position are just as serious on individuals' health as the use of tobacco.

Voilà!
30 minutes of exercise a day.
Well done!

START AN INTENSIVE WORKOUT

GOAL

Complete a physical challenge.

Have you decided that you would like to get in shape by setting a specific goal or are you already in shape and are looking for a greater challenge?

TIP

A partner is always an asset in this project. Ask for advice and look for testimonials.

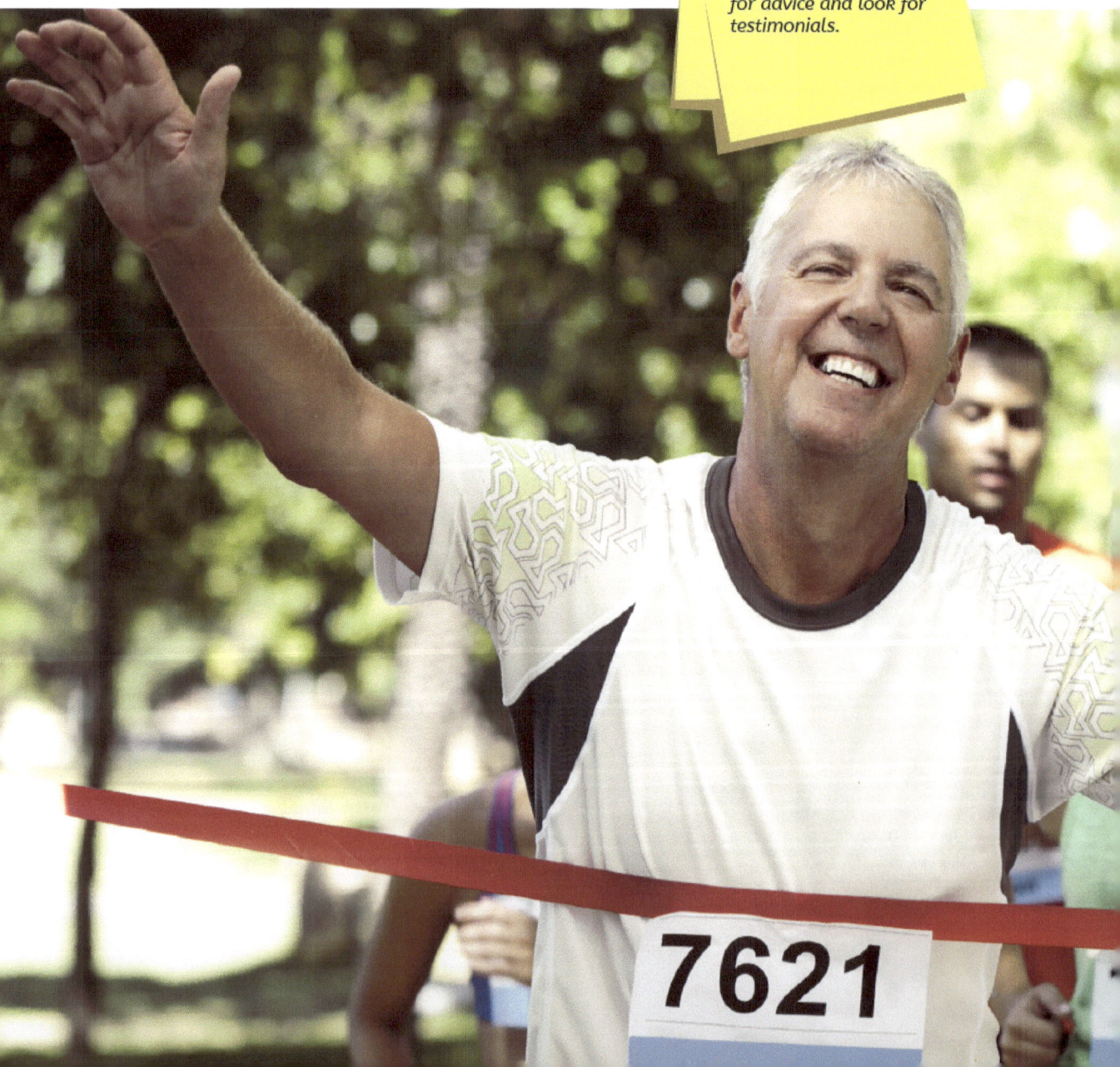

7621

HOW?

1 Determine the challenge and the date.

a. If you don't know what to choose, ask friends, colleagues, or family members that have already participated in a particular challenge.

b. You could choose according to a specific cause to support, for example a walk for breast cancer or cardiovascular disease. Many foundations hold fundraising events that offer different types and levels of challenge.

c. Choose a sport or activity that you have already done or for which you already have the skills.

2 Once the challenge has been chosen, you must prepare.

a. Leave yourself sufficient preparation time. It is better to be too prepared than to take part in the event and be unable to finish. That is very disappointing.

b. In general plan for 6 months of preparation, especially if you are currently inactive.

c. Start with a simple challenge and a reasonable distance. It is amazing to hear people declare they are going to run a marathon when they have never ran in their life and have been inactive for years. It can be possible, but risk of injury is quite high. Be logical and reasonable!

3 Create a plan and a training schedule. This calendar will replace your logbook. Try to properly record each training session and the time it took.

a. Correspond with a trainer or a specialist in the activity that you are doing. Otherwise, buying or borrowing a book, or consulting the Internet may be sufficient.

4 Start gradually and begin each training session with a warm up that includes joint rotations. Always finish with stretching; it will prevent injuries (see appendix 11 for flexibility exercises).

5 Listen to your body and always be ready to adapt. Your plan can always change.

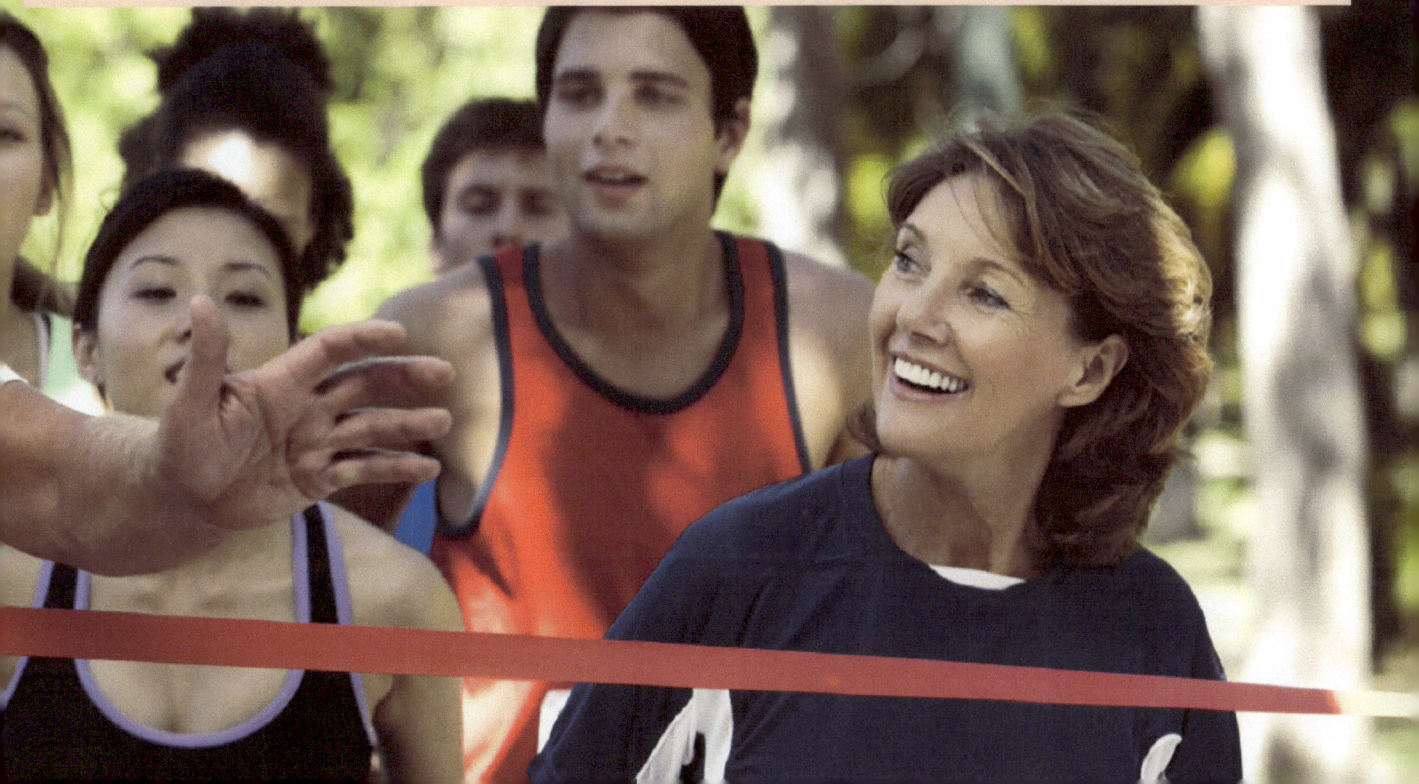

19

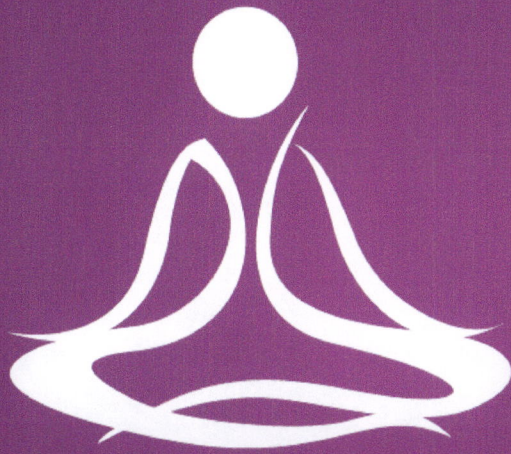

SECTION 3

STRESS MANAGEMENT AND WELLNESS

20. Practice deep abdominal breathing

21. Think of yourself

22. Plan your meals

23. Reduce daily stress

24. Get involved socially

25. Be happy

26. Stop smoking

27. Act in a civilized manner

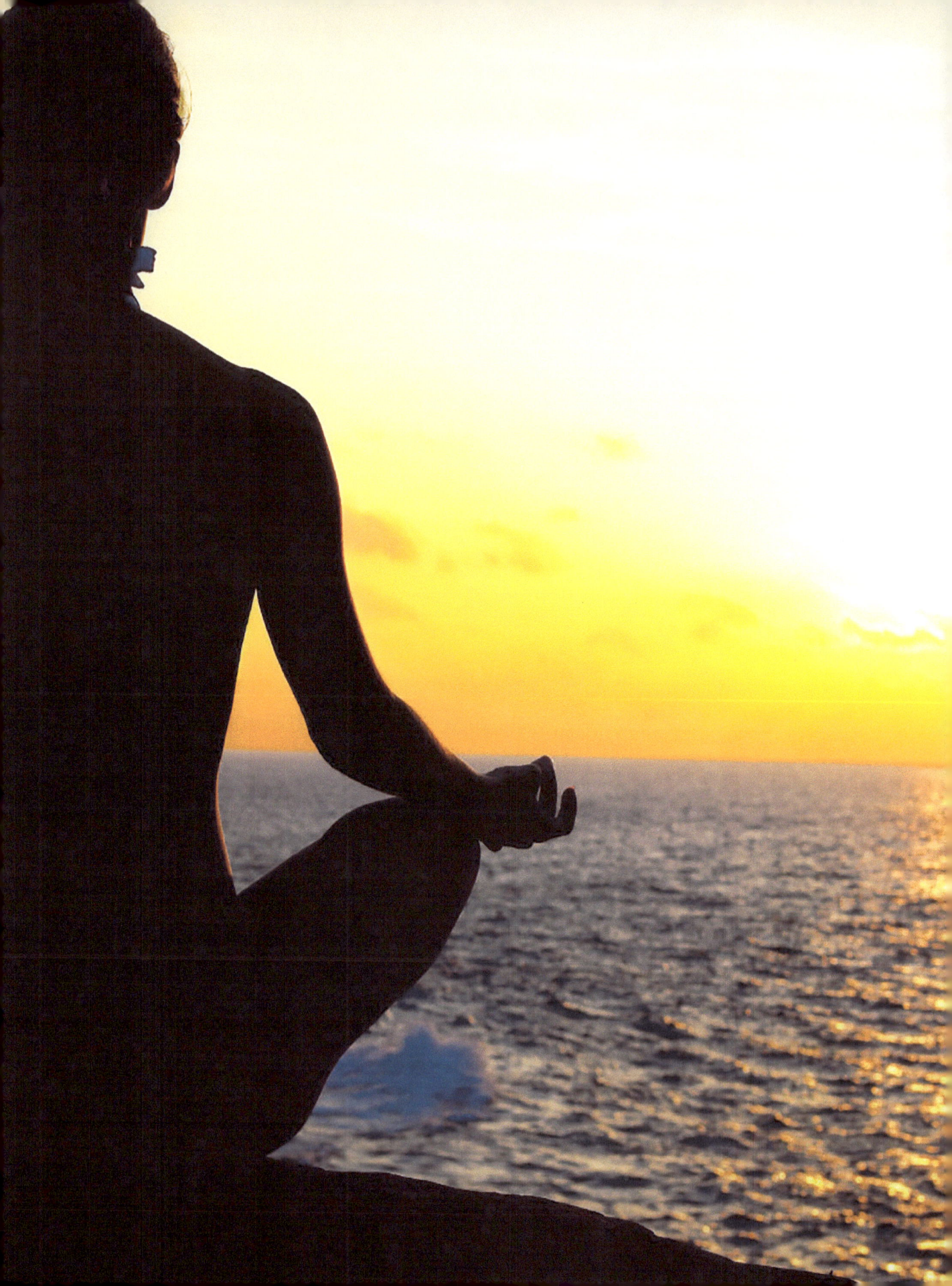

PRACTICE DEEP ABDOMINAL BREATHING

No one teaches us deep breathing, because it is assumed that everyone knows how to breathe properly. Most of us breathe in short breaths from the chest, thus preventing beneficial deep breathing. We must retrain ourselves to breathe the right way. You will find several benefits, like reduction of stress levels, better management of your mood, better blood circulation, and a general sense of well-being.

⊙ GOAL

Make deep abdominal breathing the body's automatic breathing method.

HOW?

1 Sit comfortably or lie back.

2 Inhale through the nose while trying not to inflate the chest, but the belly.

a. If you have never practiced this type of breathing, this will take you several tries to master.

3 Exhale through the mouth while pulling your stomach in towards your spine or the back of your chair.

a. This breathing method is very beneficial for stress management and during physical activity.

b. You may place your hand on your stomach to feel the inhalation and exhalation. The stomach should move up and down.

c. This breathing method should replace your current breathing method.

4 Practice this breathing method every time it comes to mind: in the car, at work, on the bus, before bed. Eventually, it will become automatic.

5 For a more relaxing or meditative version, exhale through your nose feeling the air passing through your airway and exerting pressure from the throat.

20

⚕ HEALTH INFO

Abdominal breathing improves blood circulation, increases lung capacity, and reduces the body's stress levels. During an intense moment of stress, five deep breaths can suffice in reducing perceived stress levels in the body. The Public Health Agency of Canada cites this technique as an effective method to reduce stress.

HABIT 21
THINK OF YOURSELF

Many of us live our lives at "high speed"! Between work, our kids, a spouse, family and friends, on top of the excessive amount of communications we do today, little time is left for the most important person in your life! Our lives are driven by performance and consumption. This leaves limited time to cultivate wellness, happiness, and peace of mind. The brain never has time to rest, regenerate, and clear. Work, housework, and family obligations take over, and the brain has to work three times as fast, leaving little time for peace and quiet.

🎯 GOAL

Take at least five minutes a day to relax alone or do something for yourself.

HOW?

1 Find the time to take a break, every day, at a time that suits you best.

a. Make sure the chosen moment is easy to fit into your routine.

b. Choose moments the most appropriate for your schedule and your personality.

2 Upon awakening: do five minutes of meditation while the house is still quiet.

3 In the car: If it is a long drive to work, listen to a CD with relaxing music, or a CD on an interesting subject, an audiobook...

4 If you take public transit, listen to music or read. Take this time for yourself, and do not think of it as wasted time. Take this time as a gift.

5 At work, recline your head and close your eyes for five minutes.

6 At lunchtime, take a five-minute walk (which will also be a little bit of physical activity).

7 Before going to bed, engage in an activity or hobby that you are passionate about: making models, flower decorations, sewing, do-it-yourself projects, crafts, renovations, reading, yoga, meditation, listening to music or nature sounds, a relaxing bath...

8 Complete a 21-day cycle, and then you can add more frequent or longer periods, as you see fit.

⚕ HEALTH INFO

Numerous studies have shown that relaxing activities where we are in-tune with our spirit can reduce the level of stress and increase well-being among generally healthy people. These relaxing activities can also thwart the clinical effects of stress like hypertension, anxiety, diabetes, and aging.

The four main activities recommended to reduce stress are yoga, meditation, deep breathing, and prayer.

PLAN YOUR MEALS

This habit allows you to better manage the limited time available each week and consequently, manage your stress levels too. Successfully planning your meals helps to better manage your budget and improve the quality of the family's diet since it will make you less inclined to make poor choices.

During consultations to improve lifestyle, this activity is often asked about, especially by working parents with young kids.

HOW?

1 Print the meal-planning sheet (appendix 15).

2 Establish the day that you usually do groceries.

3 Determine the meals for the next week (you can make your choices according to the weekly specials from your grocer's circular).

4 Once your meals are chosen, make your grocery list out of the necessary ingredients that you are missing.

5 You may decide to prepare certain meals over the weekend or at least prepare certain ingredients (for example, cutting vegetables, making the dressing or sauce).

6 Always plan to make a larger portion than necessary in order to have leftovers for a second meal or for lunches.

☉ GOAL

Each week, plan all meals and the grocery list.

HABIT 23
REDUCE DAILY STRESS

If you realize that you are stressed too often and you feel that your health is affected by certain symptoms (headaches, sweaty palms, stomach-aches, numbness, chest tightness, palpitations, skin irritation, back pain, musculoskeletal disorders...), it may be time to do something to lower your stress level.

⌖ GOAL

Recognize the signs of stress in the body, and perform a stress reduction technique.

! This habit will help you maintain an acceptable stress level for your health.

HEALTH INFO

- *90% of illnesses are related to stress, according to the Centre for Disease Control and Prevention (CDC).*

- *Chronic stress can reduce the effectiveness of the immune system. On the other hand, stress reduction techniques like deep breathing, meditation, and yoga, reverse this effect and increase the number of immune system cells as well as endorphins (happy hormones).*

- *Stress contributes to the development of cardiovascular diseases and to high blood pressure.*

- *Dermatologists have found that many skin irritations like eczema are related to stress.*

- *Stress is also blamed for a multitude of problems such as chronic headaches, backaches, stomach-aches, digestive disorders, insomnia and loss of sex drive.*

- *Stress stimulates the appetite and consequently, it contributes to weight gain.*

HOW?

1 Start recognizing your stress levels throughout the day by identifying symptoms.

a. Try to maintain this level between 4 and 6 (10 being the highest level of stress you could withstand).

b. Record this number in your Outlook calendar, agenda, cell phone, or logbook.

2 Recognize your physical symptoms: stomach ache, headache, sweaty palms, palpitations, increased heart rate, numbness of the extremities, digestive problems, back pain, sudden sadness, anxiety or panic attacks...

3 When you feel these physical signs, stop for a few seconds and breathe deeply 3 to 5 times, as demonstrated in habit 20. You can also take a short walk, change locations, or listen to music...

4 Calculate an average of your stress level at the end of each week. If you are regularly too high (7 to 10), you should take action and make a more significant change:

a. Speak to your supervisor or a colleague.

b. Discuss it with your spouse or a friend.

c. Try to identify the causes of your stress and act accordingly. Are you overworked, is there a conflict at work or at home?

d. Physical activity, like walking is beneficial.

e. Consult a health professional.

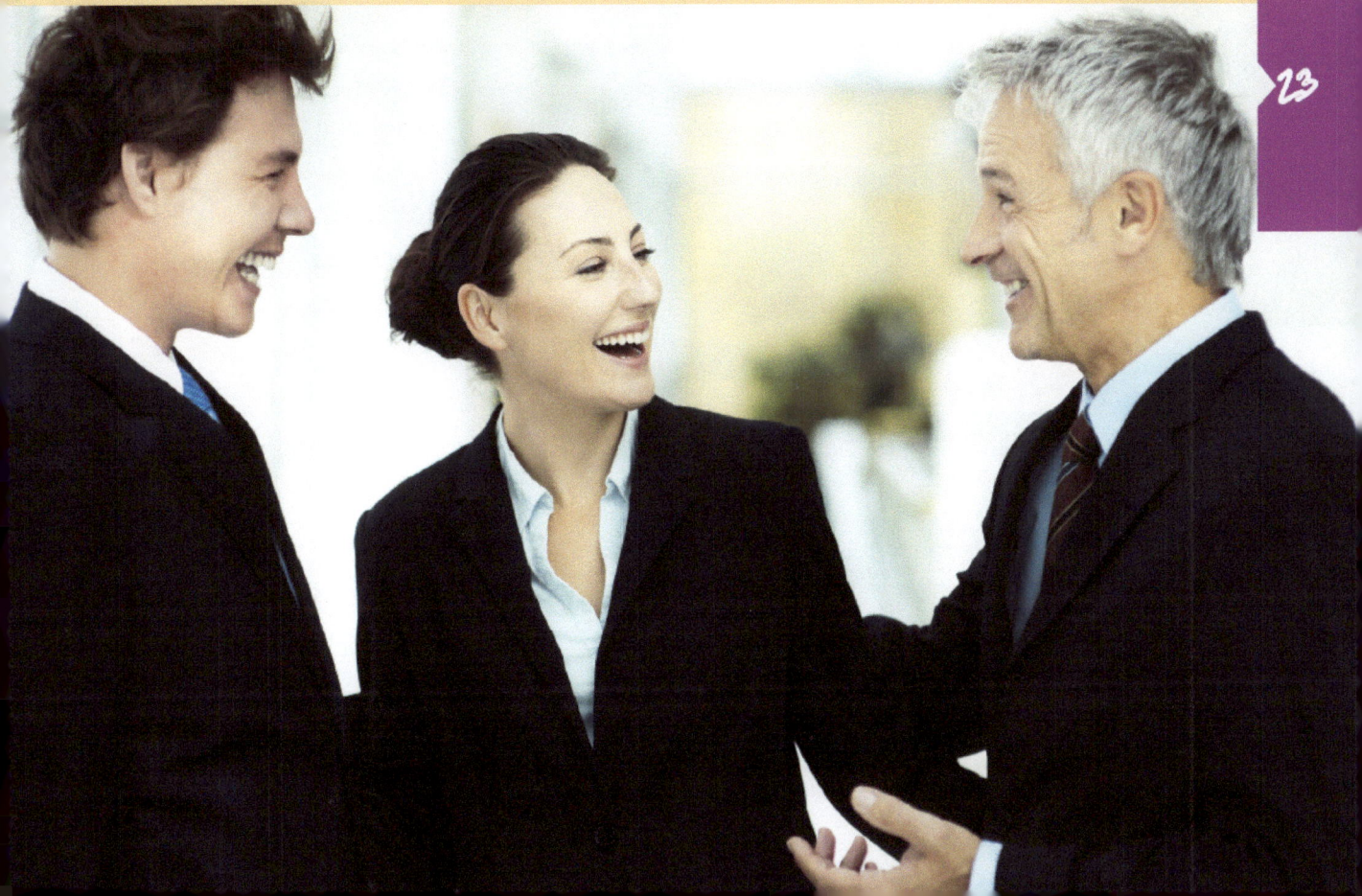

23

GET INVOLVED SOCIALLY

The more we do, the busier we are, the more efficient we become. If you have the time, getting involved in organizations that interest you – whether it's your children's school, a charity, a foundation or a cause that is dear to you – is always good for your morale.

Devote several hours a month to help out and do a good deed. It has been proven by several studies that time spent volunteering and doing good deeds is beneficial for your mental health. Moreover, several companies have already implemented programs to support the community or offer programs for a sabbatical to allow individuals to go help out in a third-world country. These experiences have proved to be a great success and people have returned refreshed, positive and very grateful.

HOW?

1 Choose your cause or organization.

2 Evaluate how much time you have to offer per week or per month (do not overload yourself).

3 Call and sign up.

4 Be careful not to do too much. The danger when we volunteer is that it can easily turn into full time work. You must always remember to think of your own well-being before all else.

☑ GOAL

Help an organization of your choice according to your availability.

HEALTH INFO

LIVE LONGER BY BECOMING A VOLUNTEER

An American study on 10,317 residents of the state of Wisconsin, since the year they graduated in 1957 until today, revealed that the most dedicated volunteers had a lower mortality rate in 2008 than people who did not engage in this sort of activity.

1 Each morning, wake up in good spirits, ready to encounter a new day. Thank life for giving you another day.

2 Appreciate what you already have. Once a week, identify at least one thing that satisfies you.

3 Live in the moment.

4 Appreciate the people you love and tell them every day.

5 Give your time.

6 Practice deep breathing, meditation, or yoga.

HABIT 25
BE HAPPY

Being happy is a good habit and a conscious decision made each day. People wait for happiness to arrive, but it is already within us and we decide, or don't decide, to live it. Most of us unfortunately don't take the time to be happy.

Happiness is within you and not to be bought: living in a bigger house, buying a new car, going on vacation – these are material goods that do not bring happiness. We must find happiness in ourselves each day. It is there, waiting. We must appreciate life. Being happy is one of the best habits that this guide can teach you. Each day, make the conscious choice to be happy. Do not wait any longer.

And if a part of your life makes you really unhappy, then you have 3 choices:

• Accept it and move on.
• Change it to make it better.
• Remove it completely from your life.

⌖ GOAL

Be aware of your happiness each day.

⚕ HEALTH INFO

A team of researchers at Harvard School of Public Health analyzed the results of more than 200 studies to evaluate the effect of psychological well-being on the heart. The results of their analysis established that happiness is a non-negligible factor toward health, reducing 50% of the risk of cardiovascular diseases despite age, socioeconomic status, smoking or weight.

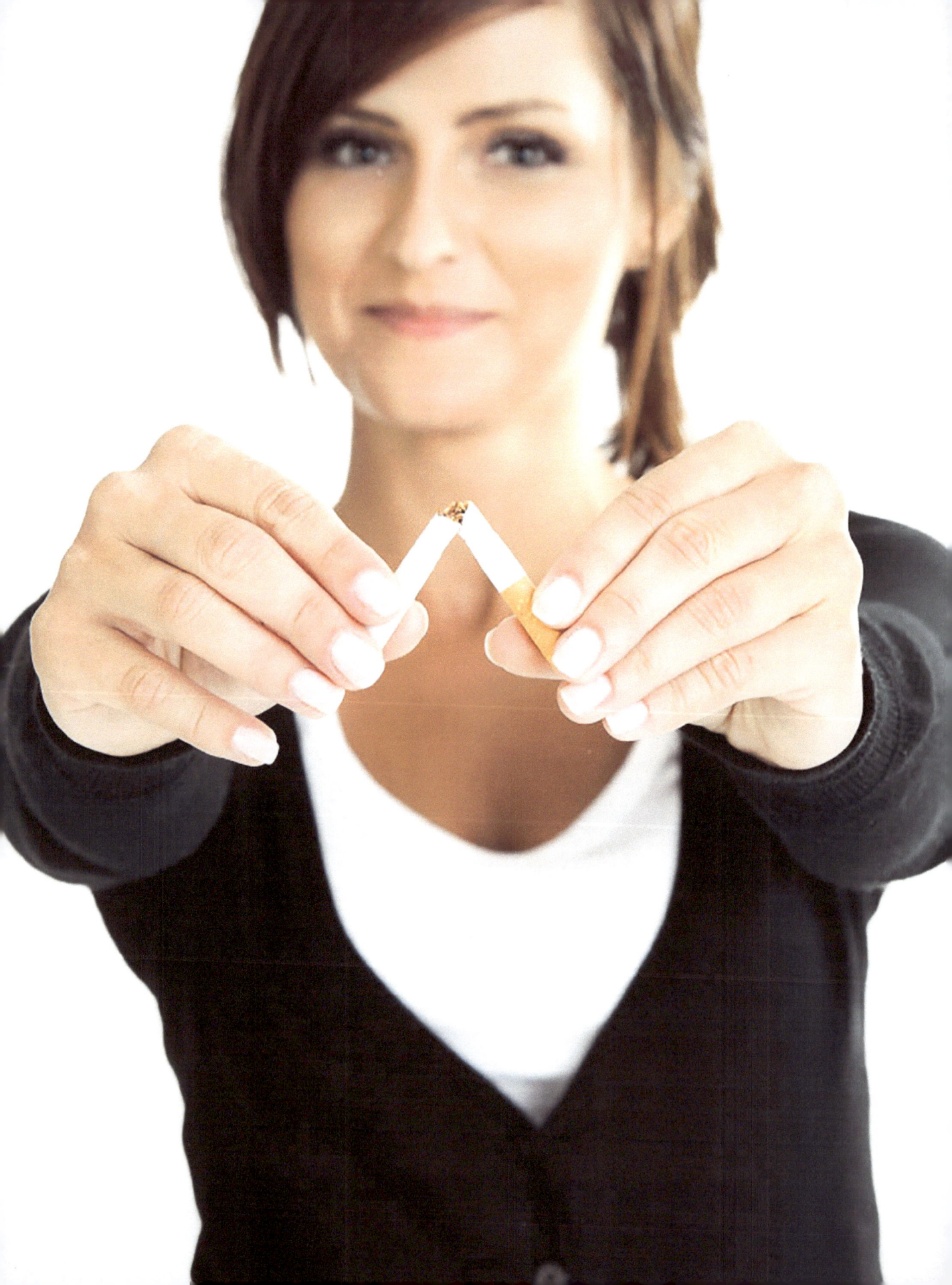

HABIT 26
STOP SMOKING

Smoking is an especially difficult habit to break, because it consists of psychosocial, addictive, and behavioural elements.

This guide will only refer to the methods and sources available in your area.

The first choice should be to consult your doctor or pharmacist. If you don't have one, you can consult your neighbourhood CLSC (for readers in Quebec) or medical clinic if you are outside Quebec. As another solution, many foundations have material resources that can help, such as The Heart and Stroke Foundation or the Canadian Cancer Society. You can visit their website or get their documentation by mail.

If you live in another country, refer to medical authorities or organizations in your region.

Quitting smoking is different for everyone. Some people do it suddenly and don't need help. Others will try ten times and experiment with every possible method with no success.

The most important thing for this bad habit will be your motivation. The Prochaska model (page 19) applies well to this situation. You may also benefit from this guide's proposed method and record the actions taken and the reasons that motivate you to stop. Find a reason to stay on track and you will persevere when the habit surfaces.

26

HEALTH INFO

STATISTICS WORLDWIDE:

- *Tobacco kills half of those that use it.*

- *The smoking epidemic kills almost 6 million people every year. More than 5 million of those are smokers or ex-smokers, and more than 600,000, non-smokers involuntarily exposed to smoke.*

- *If no urgent action is taken, the annual number of deaths could reach 8 million between now and 2030.*

- *Though it is lowering in some countries among high-income or upper-middle income, the total consumption of tobacco products are increasing at the global level.*

HABIT 27

ACT IN A CIVILIZED MANNER

The society in which we live makes us more and more selfish and self-centered. We are always in a hurry and think only of our own tasks and activities. The stress experienced every day makes us aggressive, impatient, and condescending.

Courtesy, civility, compassion, and gratitude are qualities that have almost disappeared from our daily lives.

Take the time to thank a cashier, allow a pedestrian to cross, let a car go ahead of you, help an elderly person, and lend a hand to a co-worker. Each day, do a good deed; you will see the difference in your mood and happiness.

GOAL

Do a good deed every day

HOW?

1 Identify situations when you are particularly impatient.

2 Make a list of good deeds to do.

3 Take the time to think of them each day.

4 Change your attitude toward the people you encounter.

5 Consciously decide not to transfer your stress, impatience, or bad mood onto others.

6 Do a good deed every day for 21 days.

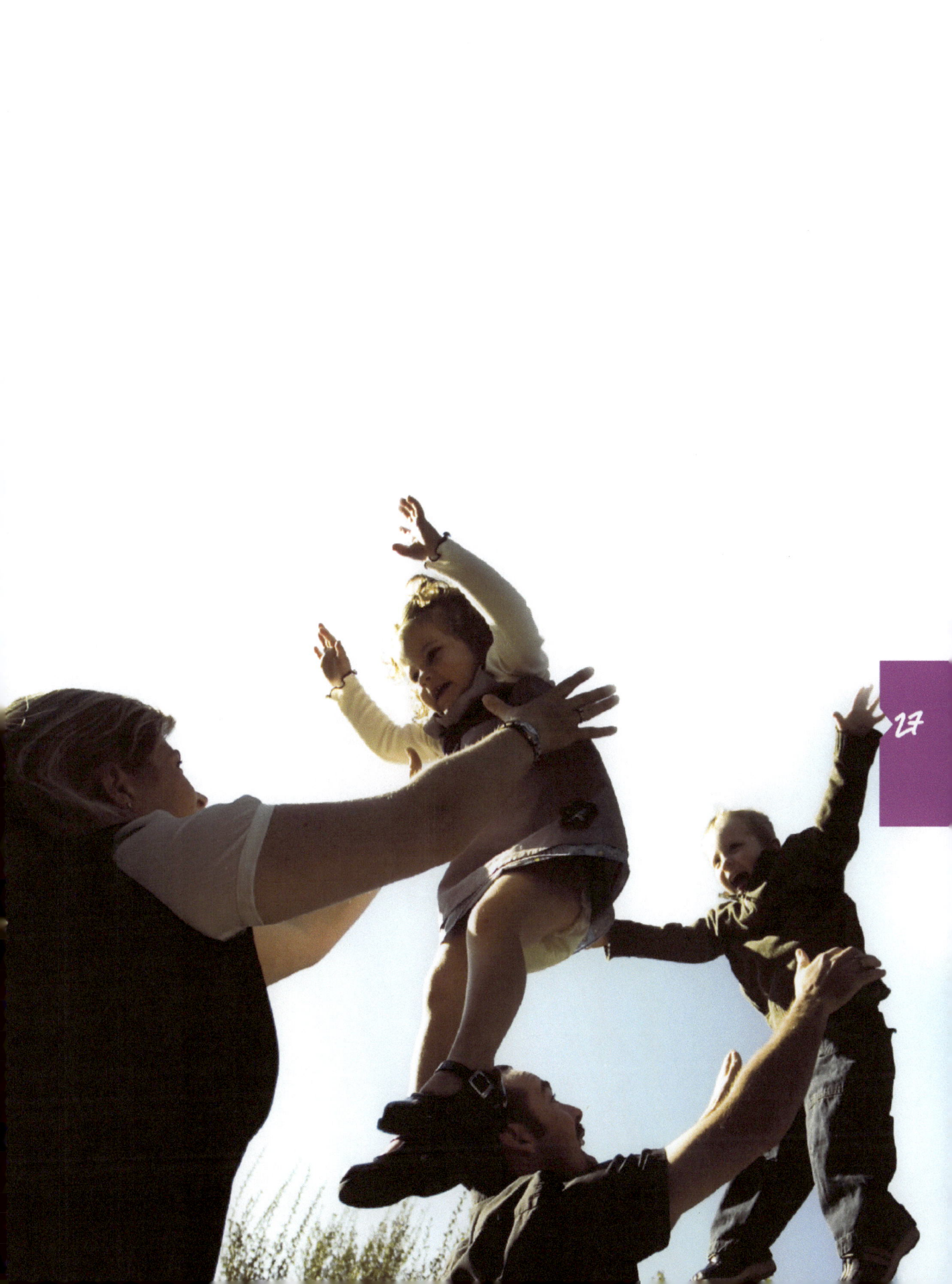

27

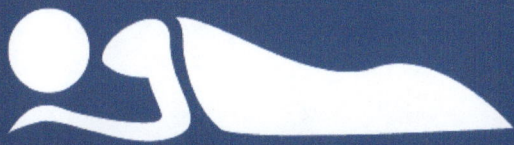

SECTION 4

SLEEP

28. Sleep more

29. Adopt a consistent bedtime routine

30. Sleep better

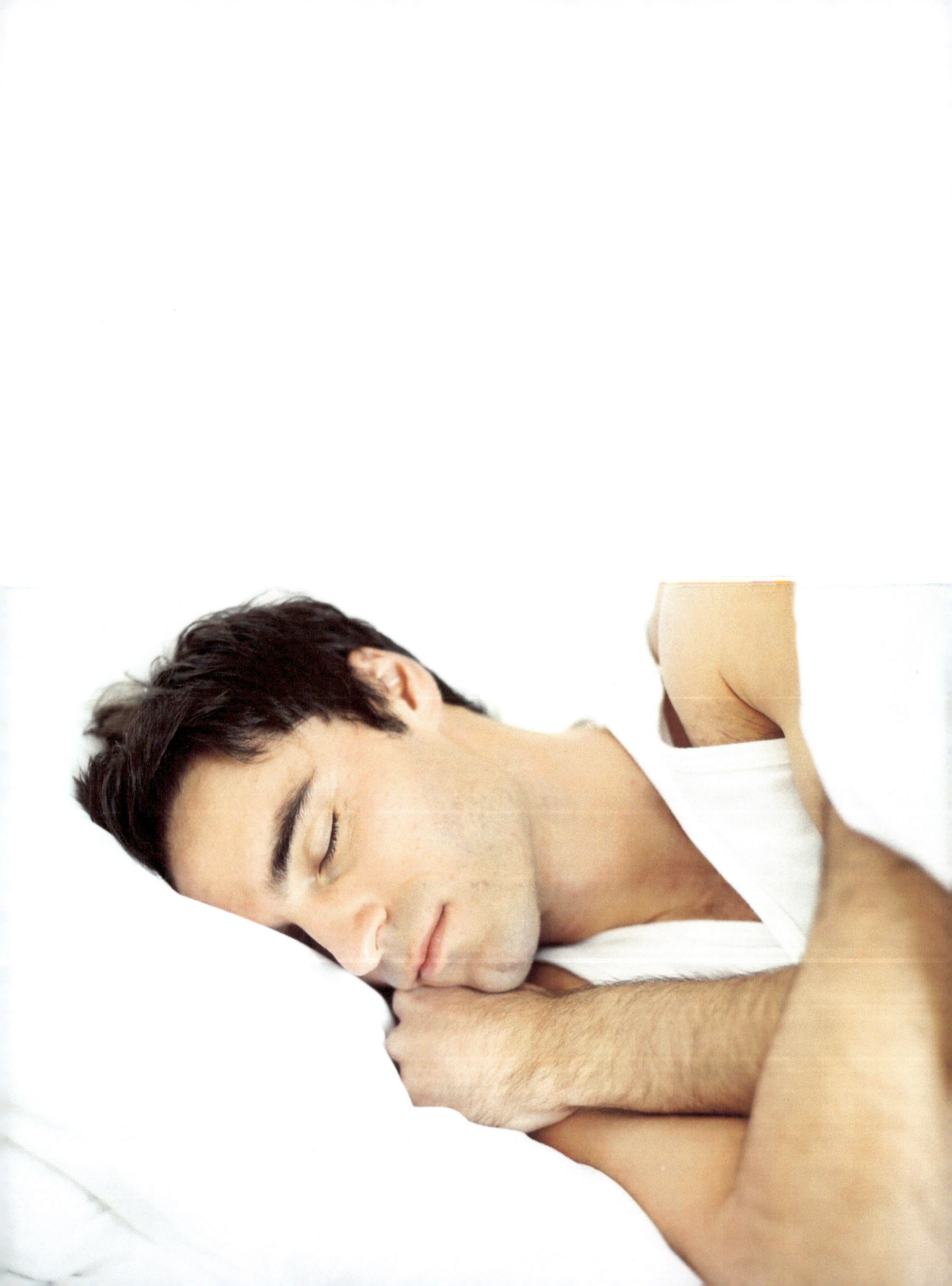

HABIT 28
SLEEP MORE

It is important to sleep between 7 and 9 hours a night. A complete night's sleep consists of 4 or 5 cycles of 1.5 or 2 hours. It is easier to wake up at the end of a cycle than in the middle. Everyone has different needs; some people function well with as little as 4 to 6 hours a night, but they are the exception (around 5% of the population). For the majority of the population, the required number of hours is 7.5 to 9.

Nighttime is when your cells replenish. It is important to our health to give them the time to do their work. A light sleep or a lack of sleep prevents the cells from regenerating.

The two most important criteria for determining if we have slept enough are:

1. Waking up well rested.
2. Functioning fully throughout the day.

⌖ GOAL
Sleeping enough to provide the body with necessary rest.

HOW?

1 Establish the ideal number of hours you feel necessary for an optimal energy level.

2 Calculate your bedtime based on when you need to wake up. For example, if you have to wake up at 6:30 am and you require 7 hours a night, you should fall asleep at 11:00 pm. The time at which you go to bed is very important. We forget to allow time to fall asleep. Often, those that are always tired lack sleep and do nothing to improve their situation. They always have something else to do and a reason to postpone their bedtime.

3 Establish a routine that will motivate you to maintain the habit of going to bed at the proper time. Allow down time for your body to slow down and your melatonin to start inducing sleep (see habit 29).

4 Record the number of hours of sleep you get each night, in your 21-day calendar. It would be opportune to leave the calendar at the side of your bed.

28

HEALTH INFO

Certain essential physiological reactions happen only when we are sleeping, for example, the secretion of growth hormone, which is typically produced early in the night during the deep sleep. When we are adults, this hormone then promotes the development of mass and muscular strength. Also, certain cells regenerate during sleep.

HABIT 29
ADOPT A CONSISTENT BEDTIME ROUTINE

Finding a sleeping routine allows you to better relax and slowly reduces your metabolism level, induces the production of melatonin, the sleep hormone.

For example, reading, relaxing music, yoga, stretching, nature sounds, meditation. All these methods can work.

⌖ GOAL

Start a healthy routine before bedtime.

HOW?

1 Establish the time at which you would like to fall asleep.

2 Determine the number of minutes (between 30 and 90 minutes) necessary to achieve a state of relaxation.

3 Review all the activities you have to do before going to bed: personal hygiene, preparation for tomorrow, and others, to allow time for relaxation.

4 Choose your relaxing activity, perhaps something different every night: reading, relaxing music, meditation, yoga or stretching...

5 Try repeating the same sequence of actions every night.

Yawning, heavy eyelids, itchy eyes, and blinking are all signs that your body is falling asleep. It is useless to anticipate them, but once these signals appear, you should not delay going to bed, otherwise sleepiness fades after 15 minutes until the next cycle, 90 minutes later.

⚕ HEALTH INFO

- *Avoid intellectual work right before bedtime.*
- *Bright lights, work, or computer games will foster difficulty sleeping. If you do need to work, lower the brightness of your screen.*
- *At least 30 minutes before bed reserve some quiet time for calm and relaxation.*
- *Establishing your own sleep routine allows you to fall asleep naturally.*
- *By closing your eyes for 5 to 20 minutes and relaxing your body, sleep will come quickly.*
- *Practice deep breathing technique.*

SLEEP BETTER

Stress levels are very harmful to the quality of sleep. The absence of a bedtime routine can reduce the quality of sleep throughout the night. Persistent personal problems, or a difficult situation encountered during the day can also contribute to a light sleep. Other problems like sleep apnea and hyperthyroidism are also common causes. If you constantly wake up feeling fatigued, there is a good chance that you don't go into a deep enough sleep.

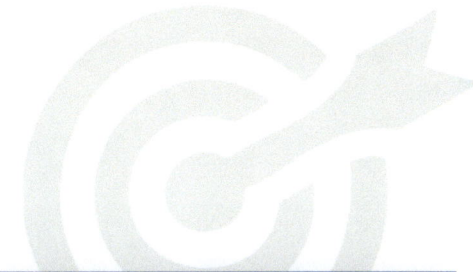

⊘ GOAL

Sleep through the night in a deep sleep, every night.

HOW?

1 See if you are stressed at the moment.

2 Keep a daily log of your sleep cycles and when you wake-up, if necessary: bedtime, times you awoke in the night, how long it took to wake up, and the time at which you got out of bed.

3 Find a solution you find effective for your situation:

a. Establish a bedtime routine.

b. Drink a herbal tea to relax.

c. Keep your linens clean and fresh.

d. Make sure that your pillow properly supports your head and that it is adapted to your sleeping position.

e. Is your spouse's snoring waking you up?

f. Modify the temperature and the darkness in your room (the sleep hormone, melatonin, is secreted in the dark).

g. Engage regularly in physical activity during the day to promote sleep.

h. Consume a dairy product, as they are recommended in the evening.

APPENDICES

APPENDIX 1
PERSONAL CONTRACT

I, _____, the undersigned, agree to take charge of my health. To do so, I agree to follow this guide and the suggested advice with the maximum effort possible. I know that these lifestyle habit changes will help me maintain better health and improve my quality of life. I also know that my lifestyle habits will have a positive impact on my own health and well-being. I make this commitment to myself and I promise to follow the "21-day" method for the following habit:

GOAL: (Write down the habit you wish to change)

_____

I will complete the logbook for the habit I chose in order to better identify the actions to take toward changing my habit.

In 21 days, on the _____ (enter the end date of your process), I will record my results.

This contract was signed on this date, _____

Participant's signature: _____

Coach/witness' signature: _____

RESULTS OBTAINED:

The habit I wish to change: _____

Have you succeeded in changing your habit within 21 days?

☐ YES   ☐ NO

If you answered yes, make sure to continue in the right direction. We must always continue to invest effort. You have moved on to the "Maintain" stage of the Prochaska model. If you answered no, identify the reasons that prevented you from reaching your goal, and restart when you are ready and you have found the motivation.

You can make a copy of this contract and display it where you can see it (on the fridge, on your bedside table, on the kitchen bulletin board, or at your desk) and/or give it to your coach to motivate you to hold your commitment.

PDF version online at aveolancis.com in the Publications section.
©AveoLancis, 2014.

CONGRATULATIONS!
YOU HAVE SIGNED YOUR CONTRACT TO TAKE CHARGE OF YOUR HEALTH!

APPENDIX 2
21-DAY LOGBOOK

IDENTIFY THE HABIT TO CHANGE: _____

TRANSFORM THE HABIT CHANGE INTO A SMART GOAL

_____

RECORD YOUR STEPS FOR SUCCESS

1. _____
2. _____
3. _____
4. _____
5. _____

CALENDAR DATES

Starting date: End date:

HABIT TO CHANGE

21 consecutive days of change (check off your success)

1	2	3	4	5	6	7	8	9	10	11	12	13	14	15	16	17	18	19	20	21

COMMITMENT:

I, _____ , agree to follow the steps and do my best to change this bad habit for 21 consecutive days, at the end of which I will allow myself to (choose a reward)

APPENDIX 3 A
LOGBOOK – EXAMPLE 1

IDENTIFY THE HABIT TO CHANGE:
Exercise daily

TRANSFORM THE HABIT CHANGE INTO A SMART GOAL
Do 30 minutes of activity at least 5 days a week for the next 21 days

RECORD YOUR STEPS FOR SUCCESS
1. *Choose the exercise*
2. *Record the time blocks in my agenda*
3. *Have the necessary equipment*
4. _____
5. _____

CALENDAR DATES
Starting date: *February 14 2014*   End date: *March 6 2014*

14	15	16	17	18	19	20	21	22	23	24	25	26	27	28	1ᵉʳ	2	3	4	5	6

HABIT TO CHANGE
Do 30 minutes of physical activity
21 consecutive days of change (check off your success)

1	2	3	4	5	6	7	8	9	10	11	12	13	14	15	16	17	18	19	20	21
√	√	√	N	√	√	√	√	√	N	N	√	√	√	√	√	√	N	√	√	√

COMMITMENT:

I, _Isabelle Lipari_ , agree to follow the steps and do my best to change this bad habit for 21 consecutive days, at the end of which I will allow myself to *a night at the movies.*

©AveoLancis, 2014.

APPENDIX 3 B
LOGBOOK – EXAMPLE 2

IDENTIFY THE HABIT TO CHANGE:
Eat more fish

TRANSFORM THE HABIT CHANGE INTO A SMART GOAL
Eat fish at least twice a week

RECORD YOUR STEPS FOR SUCCESS
1. *Find interesting recipes*
2. *Make menus in advance*
3. *Buy fresh fish*
4. _____
5. _____

CALENDAR DATES
Starting date: March 6 2014   *End date: March 26 2014*

6	7	8	9	10	11	12	13	14	15	16	17	18	19	20	21	22	23	24	25	26

HABIT TO CHANGE
Eat fish twice a week for the next 3 weeks (check off your success)

1	2	3	4	5	6	7	8	9	10	11	12	13	14	15	16	17	18	19	20	21
		√			√				√		√				√				√	

ENGAGEMENT:

I, _Nicole Lavoie_ , agree to follow the steps and do my best to change this bad habit for 21 consecutive days, at the end of which I will allow myself to *buy a new shirt.*

APPENDIX 4
SMART GOAL

A SMART GOAL
How to set a "SMART" goal and ensure success

SPECIFIC: A goal should be precise, clear, and without ambiguity.
Good Example: "Do 30 minutes of physical activity, three times a week."
Bad Example: "Do physical activity."

MEASURABLE: A goal should be measurable in order to be able to measure its progress, but doesn't necessarily require numbers.
Good Example: "Increase the amount of fruit consumed each day."
Bad Example: "Eat better each day."

ACCEPTABLE: A goal should be acceptable for people environmentally.
Good Example: "Eat 2 servings of fish per week."
Bad Example: "Eat fish every night."

REALISTIC: A goal should be realistic, in other words achieving the goal is possible in the allotted time.
Good Example: "Lose 15 lbs. in the next three months."
Bad Example: "Lose 100 lbs. in one week."

TEMPORAL: A goal should be temporal, having a set date of completion.
Good Example: "Run five kilometres in the next month."
Bad Example: "Be able to run ten kilometres."

APPENDIX 5
TABLE OF FRUITS

FRUITS	KEY INGREDIENTS	MAY HELP
Apple	Antioxidants	Diabetes and asthma
Avocado	Monounsaturated fats	High cholesterol
Banana	Potassium	High blood pressure
Blackberries	Antioxidants	Cancer and stroke
Prune	Boron (minerals)	Osteoporosis, constipation
Raspberries	Antioxidant (ellagic acid)	Cervical, esophageal, and colon cancer
Strawberries	Antioxidants	Inflammation, atherosclerosis, and tumours
Tomato	Made of 92% water	Prostate cancer, high cholesterol
Watermelon	Papain (enzyme)	Good snack to lose weight
Papaya	Vitamin A	Digestion
Peach	Soluble fibres	Immune system and infections
Pear	Bromelain (enzyme)	Constipation, high cholesterol and heart disease
Banana	Antioxidant	Digestion and blood clots
Pomegranate	Antioxidant	Blood pressure and heart health
Grapes	Antioxidants	Blood pressure and blood clots
Grapefruit	Antioxidant	Cancer and cholesterol levels
Kiwi	Vitamin C	Health of bones, teeth and cartilage
Mango	Antioxidant	Vision
Orange	Foliate	Pregnancy
Blueberries	Largest source of antioxidants	Old age
Cantaloupe	Antioxidant	Cataracts
Cherries	Antioxidant	Inflammation and arthritis
Cranberries	Antibacterial	Urinary tract infections, ulcers and kidney stones
Fig	Fibres	Heart disease
Goji berries	Several vitamins, salt and minerals and antioxidants	Diabetes and cancer

THE BEST VEGETABLES

CATEGORY A

Alfalfa sprouts
Arugula
Bean sprouts
Beet greens
Beets
Peppers
Bok Choy
Broccoli
Collard
Cabbage, Brussels sprouts
Carrots
Cauliflower
Chard
Chinese cabbage
Chive
Green cabbage
Garlic
Green Onion
Peas
Green leafy vegetables
Horseradish
Kale
Leek
Lettuce
Mustard greens
Onion
Parsley
Peppers
Pumpkin
Sauerkraut
Shallot
Snow peas
Soybeans
Spinach
Sweet potato & yam
Tomato
Cherry tomato
Green turnip
Cress
Squash

CATEGORY B

Artichoke
Artichoke Heart
Asparagus
Avocado
Celery
Chickpea
Chili pepper
Cucumber
Eggplant
Endive
Green beans
Red bean
Kohlrabi
Lemongrass
Bean lentil
White bean
Okra
Split pea
Radish
Radicchio
Rutabaga
Turnip
Zucchini

CATEGORY C

Bamboo shoot
Corn
Jicama Lettuce (iceberg)
Lima bean
Mushroom
Potato (white)
Rhubarb
Water chestnut

APPENDIX 7
TABLE OF MINERALS

MINERALS	FUNCTION	FOODS
Chrome	Required for normal insulin activity in the digestion of fats and carbohydrates	Green beans, asparagus and prunes
Selenium	Antioxidant Synthesis of thyroid hormones	Spinach, cabbage, carrots, asparagus, onions
Fluorine	Antioxidant Synthesis of thyroid hormones Proper functioning of the immune system	Tomatoes, mushrooms, red peppers, and raisins
Zinc	Necessary for normal growth and healing	Beans, nuts *Important source in meat
Cobalt	Component of vitamin B12	Meat, but mainly lentils
Copper	Needed for the synthesis of haemoglobin in the blood	Raw vegetables, beans, beets, spinach and asparagus
Manganese	Bone formation Necessary for growth Necessary for reproduction	Bananas, spinach, greens, and ginger
Iodine	Very important for the thyroid The gland regulates speed of metabolism	Bananas, spinach, greens, and ginger
Iron	Very important in the synthesis of haemoglobin in the blood	Legumes and dry fruits
Magnesium	Necessary for the proper function of neurons Constituent of several coenzymes	Raw vegetables, bananas, spinach and lentils
Chloride	Formation of the hydrochloric acid Role in balancing blood	Bread, oysters and parmesan
Sodium	Important role in the formation of neurons	Table salt
Sulphur	Component of hormones and vitamins Necessary for the production of ATP	Garlic, onions, leeks, radish, shallot and asparagus
Potassium	Formation of bones and teeth Important role in muscle contraction Forming DNA	Potatoes, bananas, Brussels sprouts, broccoli, pumpkins, chard, beets, mushrooms, melons, pears, nettles, oranges
Phosphorous	Formation of bones and teeth Important role in muscle contraction Forming DNA	Meat and fish
Calcium	Formation of bones and teeth Involved in cellular activity *Most abundant mineral in the body	Green leafy vegetables

APPENDIX 8
TABLE OF VITAMINS

VITAMINS	FUNCTIONS	EXAMPLES
A	Maintaining good overall health Good for the skin A powerful antioxidant Promotes bone growth	Orange or yellow vegetables and greens
D	Essential for the absorption of calcium and phosphorus	Fish oils, egg yokes and fortified milk
E	Plays a role in the formation of DNA Promotes healing An antioxidant	Fresh nuts, wheat germ and Green leafy vegetables
K	Important factor in blood clotting	Spinach, cauliflower, cabbage and liver
B1	Helps metabolize carbohydrates	Cereals, eggs, pork, nuts and yeast
B2	Helps metabolize carbohydrates and proteins	Beef, lamb, asparagus, peas, beets and peanuts
Niacin	Inhibits the production of cholesterol. Helps break down triacylglycerol (bad fats, LDL)	Cereals, peas, beans, nuts and fish
B6	Involved in the production of antibodies	Tomatoes, yellow corn, spinach and yogurt
B12	Important in the production of amino acids	Milk, cheese and eggs
Pantothenic acid	Synthesis of cholesterol Important factor in the energy cycle	Greens and cereals
Folic acid	Proper maintenance of lymphatic system	Green leafy vegetables, broccoli, asparagus and citrus
Biotin	Synthesis of fatty acids	Egg yoke
C	Facilitates the action of antibodies Helps healing Antioxidant Facilitates protein synthesis	Citrus, tomatoes and greens

APPENDIX 9
LOSING WEIGHT
IS MATHEMATICAL

WEIGHT LOSS

Adopting the healthy habits in this guide should lead you to a healthy weight. If weight loss is one of your goals, know that diets don't work. Many studies show that the diets publicized in various media and organizations lead to a perpetual cycle of weight loss and gain. In many cases, the weight gained after dieting is more than the weight lost in the first place. The person weighs more than she did before. What works for weight loss is a gradual change of lifestyle habits: diet, physical activity, adequate sleep, and good stress management. It is important to remember to only make changes you believe you can keep for the rest of your life. Otherwise, you risk beginning the "yo-yo" cycle of going back and forth from your desired habits to old ones. In making the changes proposed in this guide, it is highly likely that you will reach a healthy weight.

Weight loss is simply mathematics. To lose weight, you must burn more calories each day than you consume. Hence why a combination of a healthy diet and regular physical activity is ideal. It is unnecessary to count your calories every day. This practice is complicated and will only serve to discourage you. Make good, healthy choices each day and you will see the results.

Remember that as we get older, it becomes more difficult to lose weight because our metabolism slows down. Be patient and don't look at the scale too often. To give you an idea, an individual can lose between 0.2 and 0.65 kg (0.5 and 1.5 pounds) per week. The longer the weight loss period is, the more success you will have at keeping the weight off.

Here is an example:

If you want to lose 10 kilos (around 22 pounds), give yourself at least 5 to 9 months. Apply the same steps as for habits; sign the contract, find a coach, print several 21-day calendars according to the time period. You may record the number of kgs (pounds) lost each week. Don't weigh yourself more than once a week; it is useless. Always weigh yourself the same day of the week and, if possible, not Monday.

Add these optional steps: your picture and measurements, because your progress, even if it's small, will encourage you to continue.

This being said, for some people, there is often an emotional component to losing weight. In this case, making the appropriate changes is even more difficult. If this is the case for you, identify why you crave calorie rich foods. Often, it is an pent up emotion like loneliness, sadness, frustration. It will help in changing this pattern if you take the time to identify these emotions.

APPENDIX 9 – CONTINUED LOSING WEIGHT IS MATHEMATICAL

HEALTH INFO:
People that are overweight or obese are exposed to various diseases and serious conditions:

• hypertension;
• coronary heart disease;
• type 2 diabetes;
• stroke;
• disease of the gallbladder;
• osteoarthritis;
• sleep apnea and other breathing problems;
• some cancers, including breast, colon and endometrial cancer; and
  mental health problems, such as low self-esteem and depression.

Add to the list the chronic musculoskeletal disorders related to excess weight on the joints, such as back problems, and knee and ankle pains.

Public health representatives also claim:

"Avoid fad diets. Though some permit weight loss, they generally require avoiding certain types of foods and the weight lost is quickly regained when you return to a normal diet." (Health Canada in collaboration with Public Health Agency of Canada, 2013).

Physical Activity Readiness
Questionnaire - PAR-Q
(revised 2002)

PAR-Q & YOU

(A Questionnaire for People Aged 15 to 69)

Regular physical activity is fun and healthy, and increasingly more people are starting to become more active every day. Being more active is very safe for most people. However, some people should check with their doctor before they start becoming much more physically active.

If you are planning to become much more physically active than you are now, start by answering the seven questions in the box below. If you are between the ages of 15 and 69, the PAR-Q will tell you if you should check with your doctor before you start. If you are over 69 years of age, and you are not used to being very active, check with your doctor.

Common sense is your best guide when you answer these questions. Please read the questions carefully and answer each one honestly: check YES or NO.

YES	NO		
☐	☐	1.	Has your doctor ever said that you have a heart condition <u>and</u> that you should only do physical activity recommended by a doctor?
☐	☐	2.	Do you feel pain in your chest when you do physical activity?
☐	☐	3.	In the past month, have you had chest pain when you were not doing physical activity?
☐	☐	4.	Do you lose your balance because of dizziness or do you ever lose consciousness?
☐	☐	5.	Do you have a bone or joint problem (for example, back, knee or hip) that could be made worse by a change in your physical activity?
☐	☐	6.	Is your doctor currently prescribing drugs (for example, water pills) for your blood pressure or heart condition?
☐	☐	7.	Do you know of <u>any other reason</u> why you should not do physical activity?

If you answered

YES to one or more questions

Talk with your doctor by phone or in person BEFORE you start becoming much more physically active or BEFORE you have a fitness appraisal. Tell your doctor about the PAR-Q and which questions you answered YES.

- You may be able to do any activity you want — as long as you start slowly and build up gradually. Or, you may need to restrict your activities to those which are safe for you. Talk with your doctor about the kinds of activities you wish to participate in and follow his/her advice.
- Find out which community programs are safe and helpful for you.

NO to all questions

If you answered NO honestly to <u>all</u> PAR-Q questions, you can be reasonably sure that you can:

- start becoming much more physically active — begin slowly and build up gradually. This is the safest and easiest way to go.
- take part in a fitness appraisal — this is an excellent way to determine your basic fitness so that you can plan the best way for you to live actively. It is also highly recommended that you have your blood pressure evaluated. If your reading is over 144/94, talk with your doctor before you start becoming much more physically active.

DELAY BECOMING MUCH MORE ACTIVE:
- if you are not feeling well because of a temporary illness such as a cold or a fever — wait until you feel better; or
- if you are or may be pregnant — talk to your doctor before you start becoming more active.

PLEASE NOTE: If your health changes so that you then answer YES to any of the above questions, tell your fitness or health professional. Ask whether you should change your physical activity plan.

<u>Informed Use of the PAR-Q</u>: The Canadian Society for Exercise Physiology, Health Canada, and their agents assume no liability for persons who undertake physical activity, and if in doubt after completing this questionnaire, consult your doctor prior to physical activity.

No changes permitted. You are encouraged to photocopy the PAR-Q but only if you use the entire form.

NOTE: If the PAR-Q is being given to a person before he or she participates in a physical activity program or a fitness appraisal, this section may be used for legal or administrative purposes.

"I have read, understood and completed this questionnaire. Any questions I had were answered to my full satisfaction."

NAME _____

SIGNATURE _____   DATE_____

SIGNATURE OF PARENT _____   WITNESS _____
or GUARDIAN (for participants under the age of majority)

Note: This physical activity clearance is valid for a maximum of 12 months from the date it is completed and becomes invalid if your condition changes so that you would answer YES to any of the seven questions.

CSEP | SCPE

PDF online at aveolancis.com in the Publications section.

APPENDIX 11
STRETCHING PROGRAM

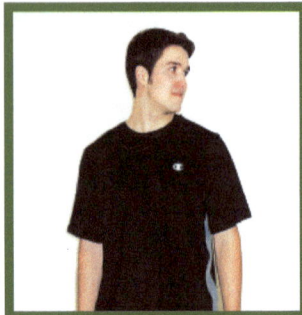

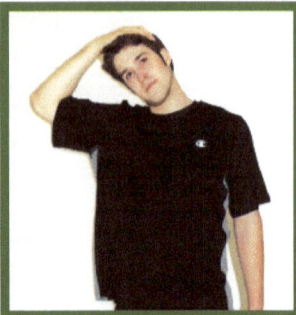

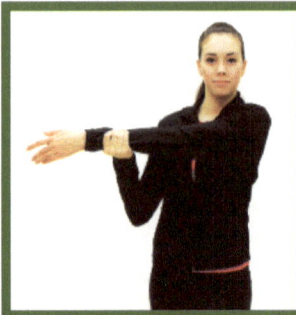

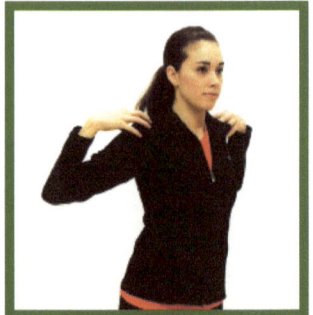

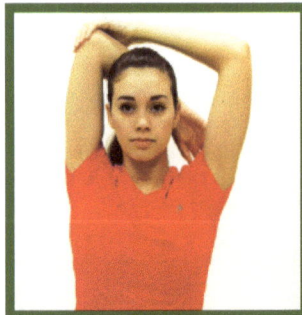

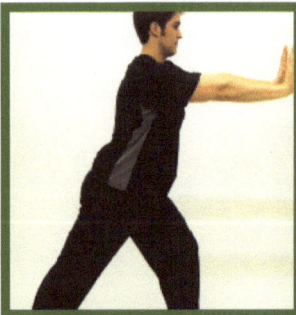

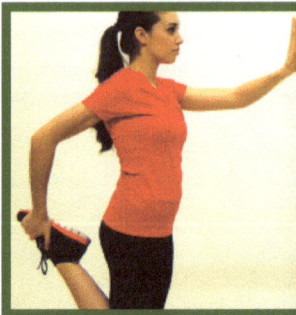

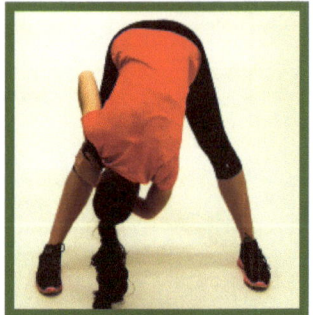

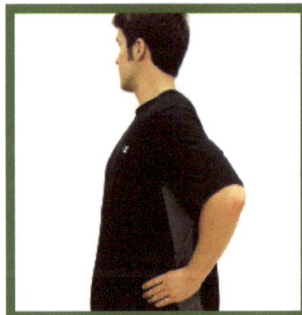

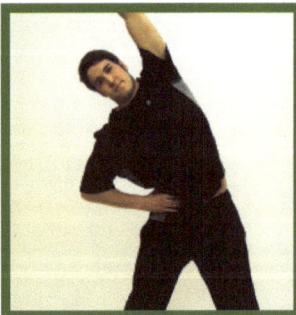

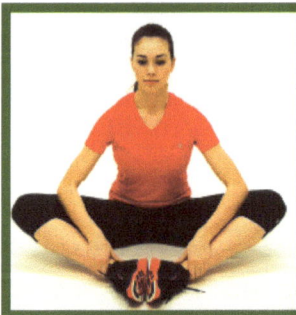

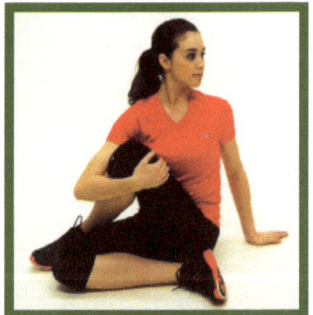

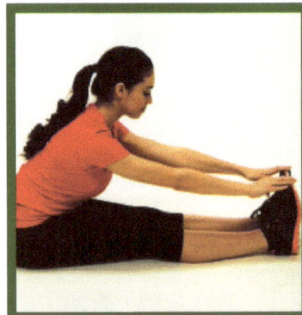

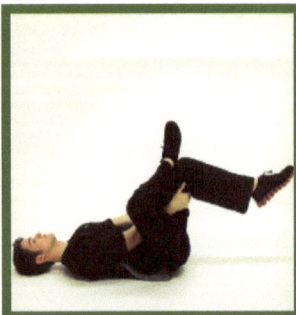

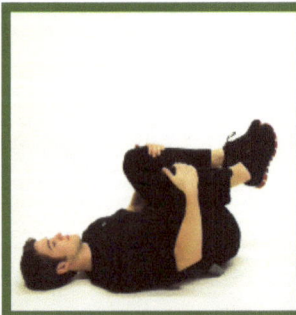

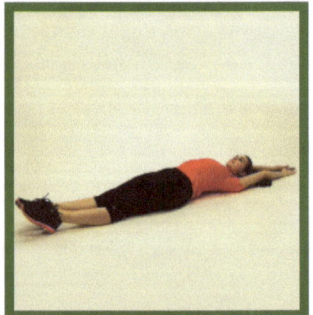

WARM-UP

Do 3 to 5 rotations of each exercise.

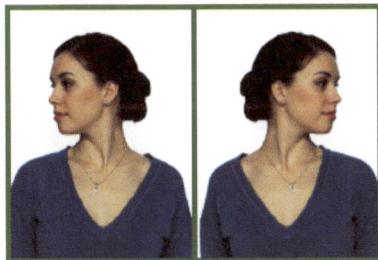

Neck side to side
Look right and left.

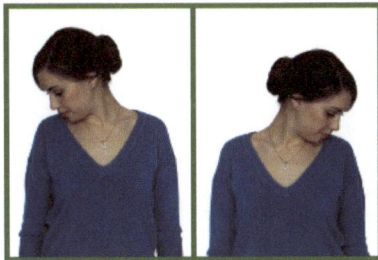

Head rotations
Be careful not to go to far back.

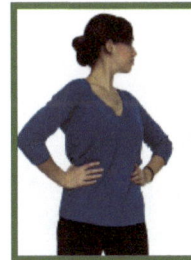

Trunk twist
With your hands on your hips,
turn your upper body to
the right and to the left.

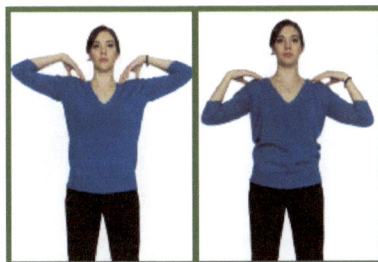

Shoulder rotations
with hands on shoulders

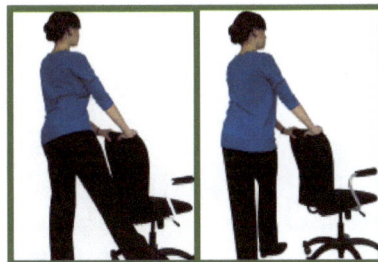

Hips
Swing each leg from side to side,
keeping hips facing front.

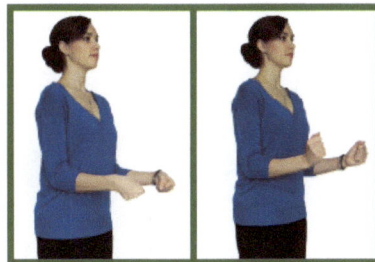

Wrist rotations

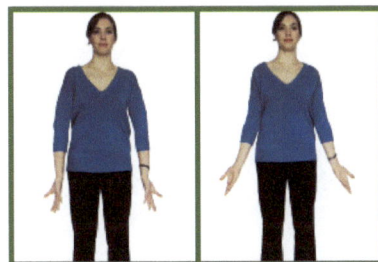

Complete twist of the
arm and wrist
Turn palms outward, then in,
rotating the whole arm.

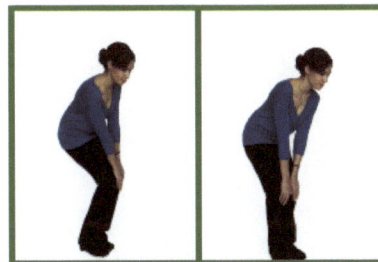

Knee rotations

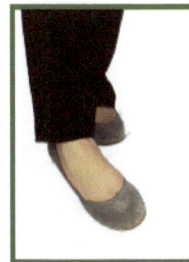

Ankle rotations
Make large circles with your foot.

STRENGTHENING
Do between 10 and 15 repetitions of each.

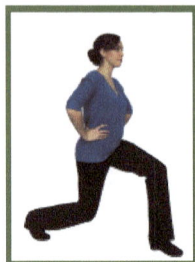

Lunge
Stepping out in front, bend your legs at a 90 degree angle.

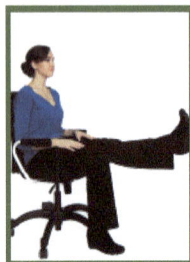

Leg extension on chair

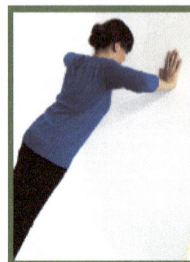

Wall push-ups
Keep your hands wider than your shoulders and your feet far from the wall.

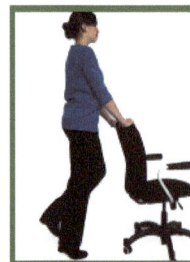

Calf rises on one leg

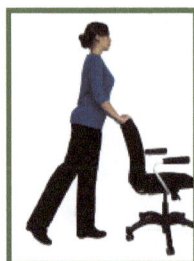

Hip extension
Lift leg towards the back, alternating each leg.

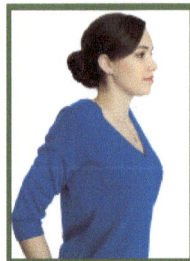

Shoulders, trapezius and back
Lift your shoulders and squeeze shoulder blades together.

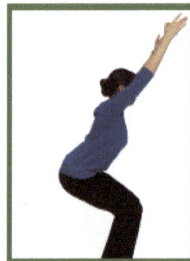

Quadriceps and core
Chair pose.

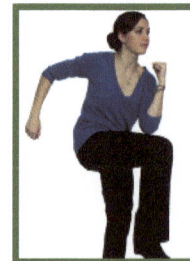

Core
Bring your elbow to your opposite knee, alternating legs.

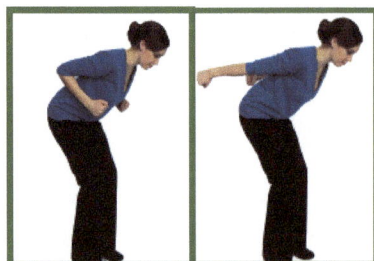

Triceps
Keeping your arms along your side and your elbows high, lift your forearm towards the back.

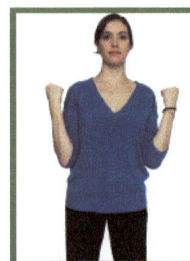

Biceps
Lift your fists toward your shoulders while keeping your arms alongside your body.

STRETCHING
Hold each stretch between 10 and 20 seconds.

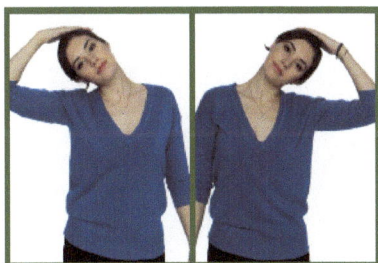

Lateral neck stretch

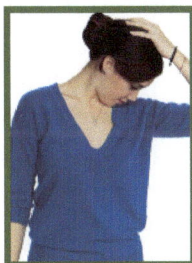

Trapezius stretch
Connect your chin to your clavicule and apply slight pressure on your head with your hand.

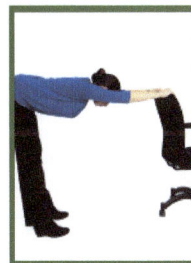

Back stretch with support

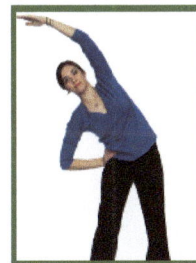

Waist and back stretch

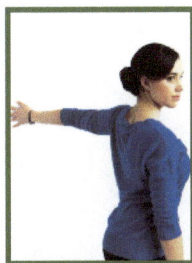

Pectoral stretch on wall
Place your palm with your thumb up on a wall, turn your body to opposite side.

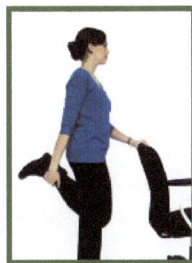

Quad stretch

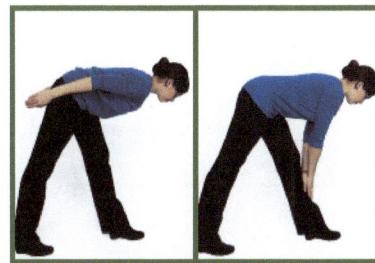

Hamstring and calf stretch

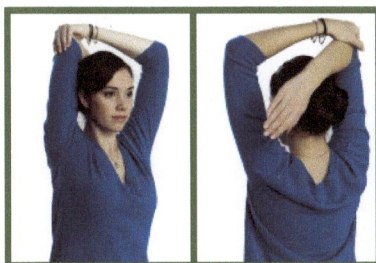

Tricep stretch

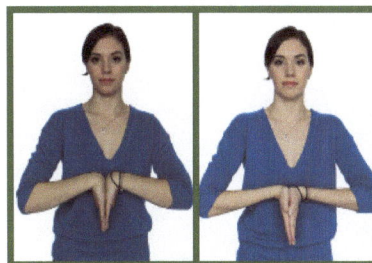

Wrist stretch
a. Back of your hands together
b. Palm of your hands together

APPENDIX 13
FATS AND OILS

TYPE OF FAT	CHARACTERISTICS	EXAMPLES	CATEGORY
Unsaturated (mono or poly)	• Healthy choices • Liquid at room temperature	• Vegetable oils (olive, canola, peanut, sesame, safflower, sunflower, corn, flax, soybean) • Avocats • Noix et graines • Poissons • Huiles de poisson	GOOD
Saturated	• Can cause diseases	• Animal meat (especially red meat) • Coconut oil • Palm oil • Dairy products (butter, cheese and whole milk) • Lard and shortening	BAD
Trans	• Even more damaging to the health	• Margarines • Fried foods • Products made from shortening or partially hydrogenated fats and oils products. (Cake, cookies, crackers, croissants...)	VERY BAD

OILS

Each oil has a different smoke point. This is the point where smoke appears upon heating the oil and when the molecular composition changes. Oils with a very high smoke point like corn oil, peanut oil, sesame oil and soybean oil are best for cooking at a high temperature. For all other medium temperature cooking, olive oil, canola oil, and grape seed oil are preferred. Avoid cooking with walnut oil or flaxseed oil because their smoke points are very low. For recipes that don't require cooking, the best choice is always olive oil.

APPENDIX 14
PAY ATTENTION
TO CARBOHYDRATES

CARBOHYDRATES

The main concept to remember about carbohydrates is that all carbohydrates are sugars. The same type of molecule can be found in a potato and in candy. Carbs are in most of our food, but in different quantities: pasta, bread, rice, fruits, vegetables, and dairy products.

There are several types of sugars, like glucose, fructose, galactose, glyceraldehyde, etc. In our foods, we can find disaccharides, a combination of two sugars. For example, a sucrose molecule (table sugar) is formed of one molecule of glucose and fructose. Moreover, there are polysaccharides, a chain of several sugars.

Carbohydrates help primarily to provide energy through the process of cell respiration. They are stored in the muscles and the liver when there is a surplus. Between carbohydrates, lipids (fats) and proteins, carbohydrates are always used first to support our body.

APPENDIX 15
MEAL-PLANNING SHEET

	Monday	Tuesday	Wednesday	Thursday	Friday	Saturday	Sunday
Dinner							
Missing ingredients							

GROCERY LIST

REFERENCES

WHY 21 DAYS?

1. "Self-Help Classics", on the Tom Butler Bowdon website, consulted November 2013, http://www.butler-bowdon. com/psychocybernets
2. Maltz, Maxwell (1960) "Psycho-Cybernetics", consulted November 2013, http://www.csi-india.org/c/ document_ library/get_file?uuid=e061fb17-048f-47e7-82f0-4341a50e07ab&groupId=47898
3. "50 Self-Help Classics", on the Tom Butler Bowdon website, consulted November 2013. http://www.butler-bowdon.com/classicslist

WHY WAS THIS GUIDE CREATED?

1.   Béliveau, Richard; Gingras, Denis (2005). Les aliments contre le cancer. Quebec : Éditions du Trécarré, 213 p.
2. Yusuf, S1. et al. (2004, Sep 11-17). "Effect of potentially modifiable risk factors associated with myocardial infarction in 52 countries" - the INTERHEART study. The Lancet 364(9438):937-52. http://www.thelancet.com/journals/lancet/article/PIIS0140-6736(04)17018-9/fulltext

WHY WAS THIS GUIDE CREATED?

1. "JAMES O. PROCHASKA, PH.D.", on the Pro-Change website, consulted January 2014. http://www. prochange.com/ staff/james_prochaska
2. Selig, Meg (2010). Changepower! 37 Secrets to Habit Change Success. United States: Routledge, 261 p.

SECTION 1

Habit 1
1. "L'eau dans l'organisme", on the National Centre for Scientific Research website. Consulted April 2013 http://www.cnrs.fr/cw/dossiers/doseau/decouv/usages/eauOrga.html
2. "Information pour les consommateurs - Innocuité des contenants en plastique d'usage courant", on the Government of Canada website. Consulted October 2013.
http://www.chemicalsubstanceschimiques.gc.ca/fact-fait/plastic-plastique-fra.php

Habit 2
"Maintenir un poids santé en mangeant des fruits et legumes", on the Government of Quebec website. Consulted October 2013.
http://www.saineshabitudesdevie.gouv.qc.ca/index.php?maintenir-un-poids-sante-en-mangeant-des-fruits-et-legumes

Habit 4
1. "Boissons gazeuses : rafraîchissantes... mais à quel prix?" on The Quebec Health and Social Services website. Consulted December 2013. http://msssa4.msss.gouv.qc.ca/fr/document/publication.nsf/ b640b2b84246d64785256b1e00640d7 4/99660f5c7b9a1db085257856006305de?OpenDocument
2. Boissons sucrées, Conséquences, "Impacts sur la santé", on the Quebec Coalition on Weight-Related Problems website. Consulted December 2013.
http://www.cqpp.qc.ca/fr/dossiers/boissons-sucrees/consequences

Habit 5
American College of Sports Medicine (2010). ACSM's Resources for the Personal Trainer. Baltimore: Lippincott Williams & Wilkins, 544 p.

Habit 6
Women's Health Magazine, March 2013.

Habit 7
"La liste noire de la malbouffe", (2009, March 19), on the website Le point.fr. Consulted September 2013. http://www.lepoint.fr/actualites-societe/2009-03-19/la-liste-noire-de-la-malbouffe/920/0/327188

Habit 8
Morissette, Claudia (2010, April 19.). "Réduire sa consommation de viande: pourquoi?", on the Passeport Santé website. Consulted September 2013. http://www.passeportsante.net/fr/actualites/dossiers/articlecomplementaire. aspx?doc=cancer_viande_rouge_et_transformee_do

Habit 9
1. Chabrillac, Odile (no date). "Manger mieux pour vivre vieux : le miracle d'Okinawa", on the Psychologies website. Consulted October 2013. http://www.psychologies.com/Nutrition/Equilibre/Regimes/Articles-et-Dossiers/Manger-mieux-pour-vivre-vieux-le-miracle-d-Okinawa/7Du-poisson-trois-fois-par-semaine
2. Sénéchal, Séverine (no date). "Prévenir par la Diète méditerranéenne", on the Séverine Sénéchal nutritional dietician website. Consulted September 2013. http://www.dieteticienne-amiens.fr/prevenir-diete-mediterranenne/
3. Coutu, Marie-France (2006, Nov. 2.). "Le poisson : plus d'avantages que de risques", on the Passeport santé website. Consulted September 2013. http://www.passeportsante.net/fr/Actualites/Nouvelles/Fiche.aspx?doc=2006110338
4. Mozaffarian D, Rimm EB (2006, 18 Oct.). "Fish Intake, Contaminants and Human Health, Evaluating the Risks and the Benefits", JAMA.

Habit 10
Asp, Karen (no date). "8 Natural Remedies That May Help You Sleep", on the Health website. Consulted September 2013. http://www.health.com/health/gallery/0,,20306715,00.html

Habit 11
1. Tortora, Gerard; Derrickson, Bryan (2007). Principals of Anatomy and Physiology. Québec: Renouveau Pédagogique Inc, 1246 p.
2. "Estimated energy requirements" on the Health Canada website. Consulted May 2014. http://www.hc-sc.gc.ca/fn-an/food-guide-aliment/basics-base/1_1_1-eng.php

Habit 12
"Calories Burned During Exercise, Activities, Sports and Work", on the NutriStrategy website. Consulted January 2013. http://www.nutristrategy.com/caloriesburned.htm

Habit 13
"Le café est-il bon pour la santé?" (2012, July 6.), On the La Presse website. Consulted January 2013. http://www. lapresse.ca/vivre/sante/nutrition/201207/06/01-4541346-le-cafe-est-il-bon-pour-la-sante-.php

SECTION 2

1. Hutton, Janice (2000). Personal Trainer Specialist Certification Manual. Ontario : Can-Fit-Pro, 265 p.
2. "Les bienfaits de la marche" (no date), on the Index santé website. Consulted September 2013. http://www.indexsante.ca/articles/article-15.html
Habit 14
"La sédentarité, une cause majeure de maladies et d'incapacités" (2002, April 4), on the World Health Organization website. Consulted November 2013. www.who.int/mediacentre/news/releases/release23/fr/#. UsxY678kK7c.email

Habitude 15
«Les bienfaits de la marche» (sans date), sur le site Index santé. Consulté en septembre 2013. http://www.indexsante.ca/articles/article-15.html

Habitude 16
Delavier, Frédéric; Clémenceau, Jean-Pierre; Gundill, Michael (2010). Delavier's Stretching Anatomy. Paris : Human Kinetics, 143 p.

Habitude 18
Hallal, Pedro et al. (2012, 18 juil.). «Global physical activity levels : surveillance progress, pitfalls, and prospects», sur le site The Lancet. Consulté en septembre 2012. http://www.thelancet.com/journals/lancet/article/PIIS0140-6736(12)60646-1/fulltext

SECTION 3

Habit 21
"Relaxation : les bienfaits du yoga, de la méditation et des activités anti-stress sur nos gènes" (2013, 12 March), on the HuffPost website. Consulted August 2013. http://www.huffingtonpost.fr/2013/05/12/relaxation-bienfaits-yoga-meditation-activites-anti-stress-genes-sante-sience_n_3228577.html

Habit 23
Burrows, Betty (no date). "How Stress Works", on the How Stuff Works website. Consulted August 2013. http://science. howstuffworks.com/life/inside-the-mind/human-brain/how-stress-works.htm

Habit 24
1. "Vivre plus longtemps en devenant bénévole" (2011, Sept. 19.), on the La Presse website. Consulted September 2013. http://www.lapresse.ca/vivre/societe/201109/19/01-4449184-vivre-plus-longtemps-en-devenant-benevole.php

2. "Benefits of Volunteering", on the Corporation for National and Community Service website. Consulted August 2013. http://www.nationalservice.gov/serve-your-community/benefits-volunteering.

Habit 25
"Positive feelings may help protect cardiovascular health" (2012, April 17.) on the Harvard School of Public Health website. Consulted January 2013. http://www.hsph.harvard.edu/news/press-releases/positive-emotions-cardiovascular-health/

Habit 26
"Tobacco", Fact-sheet N°339", (2013, July.), on the World Health Organization website. Consulted January 2013. http://www.who.int/mediacentre/factsheets/fs339/en/

SECTION 4

Habit 27
1. Allard, Sophie (2012, 28 May). "Dix vérités sur le sommeil", on the La Presse website. Consulted September 2013. http://www.lapresse.ca/vivre/sante/201205/28/01-4529161-dix-verites-sur-le-sommeil.php
2. "The Different Types of Sleep" (no date), on The Brain from Top to Bottom website. Consulted May 2014. http://thebrain.mcgill.ca/flash/d/d_11/d_11_p/d_11_p_cyc/d_11_p_cyc.html

Habit 28
"Comment mieux dormir", on the Santé médecine website. Consulted August 2013. http://sante-medecine.commentcamarche.net/faq/1397-11-conseils-pour-mieux-dormir

APPENDICES

Appendix 4
1. "Objectifs SMART", on the Coach RH website. Consulted January 2014. http://www.coach-rh.com/objectif-smart-commercial-vente.php
2. "Objectifs S.M.A.R.T", on the University of Ottawa website. Consulted January 2014. http://www.coop.uottawa.ca/fr/ fr-employer/fr-emp-smart.asp

Appendix 5
Rosenbloom, Cara (2008). "The Top 25 Healthy Fruits", on the Canadian Living website. Consulted November 2013.
http://www.canadianliving.com/health/nutrition/top_25_healthy_fruits_blueberries_apples_cherries_bananas_ and_21_more_healthy_picks.php

Appendix 7 and 8
Tortora, Gerard; Derrickson, Bryan (2007). Principals of Anatomy and Physiology. Québec: Renouveau Pédagogique Inc, 1246 p.

Appendix 9
Health Canada (2006). "Obésité, votre santé et vous" on the Health Canada website. Consulted December 2013.
http://www.hc-sc.gc.ca/hl-vs/iyh-vsv/life-vie/obes-fra.php

Appendix 13 and 15
Reece, Jane et al. (c2011). Campbell Biology. United States : Pearson, 1263 p.

Appendix 14
Nelson, Jennifer (2013, March 13). "Which type of oil should I use for cooking with high heat? on the Mayo Clinic website. Consulted October 2013.
http://www.mayoclinic.com/health/cooking-oil/AN02199

WORKS CITED

1.   Ledoux, Marielle; Lacombe, Natalie; St-Martin, Geneviève (2006). Nutrition Sport et Performance. Quebec : Géo Plein Air, 255 p.

2.   Huot, Isabelle; Lavigueur, Josée; Bourgeois, Guy (2008). Kilo Cardio 1. Quebec: Les éditions de l'homme, 203 p.

3.   Blahnik, Jay (2011). Full-Body Flexibility. Human Kinetics, 255 p.

4.   Reece, Jane et al. (c2011). Campbell Biology. United States : Pearson, 1263 p.

5.   Tortora, Gerard; Derrickson, Bryan (2007). Principes d'anatomie et de physiologie. Quebec: Renouveau Pédagogique Inc, 1246 p.

6.   Béliveau, Richard; Gingras, Denis (2005). Les aliments contre le cancer. Quebec: Éditions du Trécarré, 213 p.

PERSONAL NOTES